LASER ANGIOPLASTY

LASER ANGIOPLASTY

Edited by

Timothy A. Sanborn, M.D.
Associate Professor of Medicine
Director, Interventional Cardiology Research
and Laser Angioplasty Program
The Department of Medicine
Division of Cardiology
Mount Sinai Medical Center
New York, New York

ALAN R. LISS, INC. • NEW YORK

Address all Inquiries to the Publisher
Alan R. Liss, Inc., 41 East 11th Street, New York, NY 10003

While the authors, editors, and publisher believe that drug selection and dosage and the specifications and usage of equipment and devices, as set forth in this book, are in accord with current recommendations and practice at the time of publication, they accept no legal responsibility for any errors or omissions, and make no warranty, express or implied, with respect to material contained herein. In view of ongoing research, equipment modifications, changes in governmental regulations and the constant flow of information relating to drug therapy, drug reactions and the use of equipment and devices, the reader is urged to review and evaluate the information provided in the package insert or instructions for each drug, piece of equipment or device for, among other things, any changes in the instructions or indications of dosage or usage and for added warnings and precautions.

Library of Congress Cataloging-in-Publication Data

Sanborn, Timothy A.
    Laser angioplasty.
    Includes bibliographies and index.
    1. Laser angioplasty. I. Title. [DNIM:
1. Angioplasty, Transluminal. 2. Coronary
Disease—therapy. 3. Lasers—therapeutic use.
WC 166 S198L].
RD598.5.S26 1989   617′.413059   88-27214
ISBN 0-8451-4280-1

Cover: Angiograms of a twelve cm right superficial femoral artery occlusion (left panel, between black arrows) in a gentleman with one-half block claudication. Due to the hard fibrotic calcified nature of this lesion (middle panel, open arrow), this lesion could not be recanalized by conventional guidewires despite catheter support. A 2.0mm-Plus™ laserprobe easily recanalized this lesion with 10 watts of argon laser energy (middle panel). An excellent angiographic result was obtained after subsequent balloon angioplasty with a 6mm balloon angioplasty catheter (right panel).

Contents

v

Contributors

George S. Abela, Division of Cardiology, University of Florida, Gainesville, FL 32610 [47]

Gérald Barbeau, Division of Cardiology, University of Florida, Gainesville, FL 32610 [47]

Anna M. Belli, Department of Radiology, Northern General Hospital, Sheffield S57 AU, England [35]

Robert J. Bowes, Department of Radiology, Northern General Hospital, Sheffield S57 AU, England [35]

John R. Crew, Department of Vascular Surgery, San Francisco Heart Institute, Seton Medical Center, Daly City, CA 94015 [35]

David C. Cumberland, Department of Radiology, Northern General Hospital, Sheffield S57 AU, England [35]

Edward B. Diethrich, Arizona Heart Institute and the Department of Cardiovascular Services, Humana Hospital–Phoenix, Phoenix, AZ 85064 [77]

Alan J. Greenfield, Department of Radiology, Boston University Medical Center, Boxton, MA 02118 [15]

Jonathan L. Halperin, Cardiology Division, Mount Sinai Medical Center, New York, NY 10029 [7]

D. Richard Leachman, Department of Adult Cardiology, Texas Heart Institute, Houston, TX 77030 [59]

Harold A. Mitty, Department of Radiology, Director of Interventional Radiology, The Mount Sinai School of Medicine of the City University of New York, New York, NY 10029 [ix]

Richard K. Myler, Department of Cardiology, San Francisco Heart Institute, Seton Medical Center, Daly City, CA 94015 [35]

Timothy A. Sanborn, Division of Cardiology, Mount Sinai Medical Center, New York, NY 10029 [xi, 1, 21, 29, 93, 101, 111]

James M. Seeger, Department of Surgery, University of Florida and Veterans Administration Medical Center, Gainesville, FL 32610 [47]

Simon H. Stertzer, Department of Cardiology, San Francisco Heart Institute, Seton Medical Center, Daly City, CA 94015 [35]

Christopher L. Welsh, Department of Surgery, Northern General Hospital, Sheffield S57 AU, England [35]

Foreword

The growth of nonsurgical intervention as a medical subspecialty has paralleled technical developments in needle, guidewire, and catheter design. The pioneering work of Dr. Charles Dotter began the era of vessel recanalization or angioplasty with a coaxial catheter system. Cardiologists dealing with the problem of coronary atherosclerosis were interested in possible nonsurgical methods of patient management. It was at this point that Dr. Andreas Grüntzig developed the first practical balloon dilating catheter. This was used in the "safer" peripheral circulation to gain experience before its coronary applications were realized. Balloon catheters are also used outside the vascular system to dilate access tracts as well as in the treatment of a variety of strictures in the urinary and biliary tracts.

Early clinical reports of the usefulness of balloon angioplasty were followed by disappointing restenosis rates, particularly in small, diffusely diseased vessels like the superficial femoral artery. Although there have been improvements in guidewire and balloon design, the basic problem of recurrence of disease continues to plague patients and interventionalists alike. When there is no right answer to a problem there are often attempts at various solutions. It is therefore not surprising that there have been unprecedented numbers of new devices designed to solve problems associated with obliterative atherosclerotic diseases, particularly in the legs and the coronary circulation. High-speed and low-speed rotational devices, atherectomy catheters, angioscopes, and an array of different laser systems now confront the interventionalist. Hardly a week goes by that a new device is not introduced or that one recently introduced is not modified.

This book squarely attacks some of the confusion by discussing availability, techniques, and results of primary laser recanalization and the laser as an adjunct to balloon angioplasty. Early clinical results in the legs and the coronary circulation are presented.

Which laser system is best? This question is difficult to answer, as the devices are in a rapid state of change and many are in pre-market evaluation. Interventionalists must ask themselves a variety of questions before deciding to purchase a laser. Do they have case material? Is the technical and clinical expertise necessary for proper management of this group of patients available at their institutions? Are there adequate radiologic facilities to provide proper catheter guidance and imaging?

The performance of peripheral angioplasty has traditionally been in the domain of the interventional radiologist. Other interventionalists, most notably cardiologists skilled in coronary angioplasty, have a role to play. Thus, a laser can have dual functions in both radiology and cardiac catheterization rooms. The expertise of both groups can be used to the benefit of the patient. Some of the gothic stories of turf battles are undoubtedly true; each institution must solve these issues in a manner that will deliver the best patient care. It makes no sense for a vascular surgeon with no catheterization experience to spend hundreds of thousands of dollars on x-ray equipment and lasers when there are competent skilled interventionalists present in the institution's radiology department. By the same token, the patient may be served best by a combined surgical-radiologic procedure. Cooperation and the addition of skills from both disciplines provides optimal care.

One of the more disturbing aspects of the recent availability of an FDA approved laser system for angioplasty is the marketing "hype" from media and commercial sources. Hospital administrations are urging radiologists and cardiologists to acquire lasers so that their hospital can be first in the area with this new device. They argue that the resulting publicity can increase occupancy rates. Another motivation from hospital administrations has been the hope that patients admitted for therapy of peripheral vascular disease under the appropriate DRG (diagnostic related group) can be discharged earlier (having avoided the longer stay associated with surgery), resulting in a "profit" from not fully using the allotted time. Physicians must maintain perspective under these extraneous pressures and be guided by medical indications rather than economic considerations.

What does the laser do that is useful? Is it better than balloon angioplasty alone? Early responses to these questions appear in this book, which is an attempt to shed light (pun intended) on this relatively new field. The contributors are the experts in a field that is evolving rapidly. Some of their early results are encouraging; nevertheless, greater clinical experience with controlled trials will be necessary before adequate answers to these questions are obtained. In addition, we are still at a very early stage in technological development, so that many of the current reports will be in the category of feasibility studies when newer guidance and laser delivery systems are available.

Harold A. Mitty, M.D.

Preface

In the past few years, the cardiovascular application of lasers has captured the imagination of the media, the lay public, and the medical community in general. There are several laser devices that are in various stages of clinical investigation for treatment of peripheral and coronary arteries. Several such devices have been approved by the FDA for use in peripheral arteries. For the practicing radiologist, cardiologist, or vascular surgeon who is interested in learning more about this new approach, there are only a few published clinical reports to read and review. Moreover, didactic lectures or videotapes fail to describe fully the intricacies of these clinical laser procedures.

While there are some textbooks and monographs that deal with basic aspects of laser physics and laser-tissue interactions, very little has been written on clinical techniques and procedures. Thus, the present volume was organized to provide the reader with knowledge of current laser angioplasty experience and to serve as a basic "how-to" handbook of at least one laser angioplasty approach—laser thermal angioplasty with the laserprobe device. Obviously, laser angioplasty is only in its infancy, and both equipment and technique will change considerably in the next few years. This volume provides an introduction to the clinical use of lasers in cardiovascular disease.

Timothy A. Sanborn, M.D.

1. Early Results of Laser Angioplasty Using Bare Fiberoptics

Timothy A. Sanborn, M.D.

THE POTENTIAL

By partially removing obstructing atheroma or thrombus through vaporization of tissue and leaving behind a smoother luminal surface than the fracture and dissection noted with conventional balloon angioplasty [1], laser angioplasty or laser recanalization has the potential to serve as an aid or possibly as an alternative to conventional balloon angioplasty by 1) increasing the initial success rate for lesions that are difficult or impossible to treat by conventional means or 2) decreasing the incidence of restenosis.

However, in initial experimental studies and early clinical trials with bare argon laser fiberoptics, the technique was limited by inadequate delivery systems, resulting in an unacceptable high perforation rate [2–6] and the creation of small recanalized channels that resulted in poor long-term patency [4]. The key limitation in these early trials of laser angioplasty was the lack of an adequate catheter delivery system for safe and effective intravascular use of laser energy. In this chapter, basic laser properties will be briefly reviewed and the initial experimental and clinical results with bare laser fiberoptics will be summarized.

LASER FUNDAMENTALS

The Laser Process

The term laser is an acronym composed of the first letters of the words *l*ight *a*mplification by *s*timulated emission of *r*adiation. The simplest way to understand how a laser works is to visualize an active medium of atoms, molecules, and ions contained in a long cylindrical laser tube or cavity (Fig. 1–1). These atoms have the capacity to rise from a ground state to an "excited" state by absorbing energy and also to return back to the ground state by spontaneously emitting a quantity of energy in the form of light photons (Fig. 1–2). This "spontaneous emission" of light radiation spreads in all directions in the laser cavity. Although a small number of spontaneously emitted photons can travel in one direction along the length of the laser tube, the majority of the energy is dissipated in the form of heat. Thus, spontaneous emission of radiation alone does not produce a very powerful beam of light photons.

The key to the laser process is the *stimulated emission* of *radiation* in which a photon of light collides with an excited atom and the collision produces two photons of a single wavelength (monochromatic) traveling in the same direction (Fig. 1–2). These photons will collide with additional excited atoms, and more energy will develop in the laser cavity. As stimulated emission of laser action continues, atoms are removed from the upper excited state and the population of atoms in the lower ground state increases. If allowed to continue, in time, there will be a greater percentage of atoms in the ground state than in the excited state and the probability of a photon being absorbed will increase while the probability of stimulating further radiation will decrease and the laser action will cease. In order to prevent the laser action of the active medium from terminating, a process is

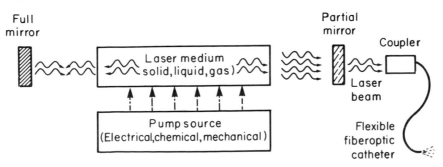

Fig. 1–1. Basic components of a cardiovascular laser device.

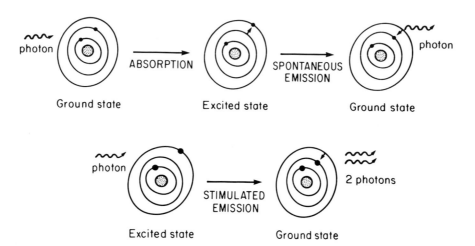

Fig. 1–2. The laser phenomenon. (Top) Absorption of a photon results in excitation of an atom from the ground to the excited state. Spontaneous emission of a photon results in the return of the atom to the ground state. (Bottom) Stimulated emission occurs when a photon encounters an atom in the excited state; the atom returns to a lower energy level, and a second photon is emitted with the same energy, wavelength, and direction as the incidence photon.

required to "pump" atoms from the lower ground state to the higher excited state. This process is called pumping and requires a source of external energy (pump source: electrical, chemical, or mechanical) that can be injected to the laser system (Fig. 1–1).

The intensity of the intracavity energy is *amplified* by multiple reflections between parallel mirrors at each end of the laser tube. At the rear end of the laser tube is a totally reflective mirror that bounces the light back down the tube. At the front end of the laser tube is a partially transparent mirror that allows a portion of the laser energy to be admitted as a narrow laser beam. This laser beam is much more powerful than ordinary light because it is *unidirectional,* traveling in a single path.

Laser Temporal Modes

Most lasers can operate in a variety of temporal modes that differ in their output with respect to time. The two major modes are continuous and pulsed. In the continuous wave (CW) mode, the laser is operating continuously, delivering laser energy as long as the operator opens a shutter by depressing a foot pedal or switch. CW output can also be divided into short repetitive bursts (0.5–5 s) or steady firing (>5 s). In contrast, with the CW laser, there is a family of pulsed lasers that generally have a pulse duration that is much shorter than that of a CW laser device (1×10^{-12} to 1×0.5 s). These pulsed lasers are able to obtain power levels that are significantly higher than those of CW devices even though they may have the same active media and may have the same laser wavelength. Thus, cardiovas-

cular lasers may vary in their temporal mode as well as in their wavelength (Table 1–1).

Laser-tissue Interactions

The actual effects of lasers on biological tissue is dependent on a number of factors including the laser wavelength (nm), pulse duration (s), power (W), and beam size (cm^2); the absorption characteristics of the tissue; and the thermal diffusion capacity ("cooling") of surrounding tissue and convective systems (blood and lymph). Laser-tissue interactions are quantitated by calculating the amount of energy distributed to the tissue. This energy is referred to as the power density or energy fluence and is described as follows:

Energy fluence (J/cm^2)
$$= \frac{\text{laser power output (W)} \times \text{exposure times (s)}}{\text{laser beam cross-sectional area (} cm^2 \text{)}}$$

However, for laser angioplasty, the fact that the fiberoptic tip is positioned in flowing blood or in contact with heterogenous human atherosclerotic lesions that change significantly after laser radiation makes mathematical calculation of laser-tissue interaction extremely complex if not impossible.

EARLY CLINICAL CARDIOVASCULAR LASER STUDIES

Although the concept of laser angioplasty is relatively new in cardiology, there already is a tremendous variety

TABLE 1–1. Characteristics of Current Clinical Cardiovascular Lasers

	Lasers			
	Excimer	Argon	Nd:YAG	CO_2
Laser				
characteristics				
Spectral region	Ultraviolet	Visible	Near infrared	Infrared
Wavelength (nm)	308	488,514	1,060	10,600
Temporal mode	Pulsed (P)	CW	P, CW	CW
Delivery systems	Fiberoptic	Fiberoptic; metal cap; combined metal cap-sapphire tip; lensed tip	Fiberoptic; metal cap; sapphire tip; laser-balloon	Rigid instrument
Pathophysiological				
mechanisms				
Vaporization	+	+	+	+
Thermal compression	−	+	+	−
Sealing	−	−	+	−

of different laser approaches in the various stages of experimental and clinical investigations (Table 1–1). These clinical cardiovascular laser systems are often separated by their laser wavelength (argon, Nd:YAG, CO_2, excimer, etc.); however, each laser has the potential to be used with a variety of different delivery systems, some of which can be interchanged with other laser generators. In the future, the clinical success of a laser angioplasty system may depend more on the specifics of the individual fiberoptic delivery system and the pathophysiological mechanisms of action of lasers (Table 1–1) than on the actual laser generator itself.

Bare Argon Laser Fiberoptics

The argon gas laser was the first to be used experimentally [7–11] and clinically [5,6] for laser angioplasty. Rather than any particular characteristic of laser wavelength or other physical properties, this early use was more related to its availability from other medical applications and the fact that the visible argon light is readily transmitted by glass optical fibers. Thus, the argon laser had already been used extensively in other areas of medicine and the laser system was already well developed.

Laser properties. The argon laser operates in a CW mode, and the laser generator is capable of delivering up to 20 W of power. The wavelengths most commonly used for medical application are in the blue-green spectral region at 488 and 514 nm. This blue-green light is readily absorbed by chromogens in the arterial wall and hemoglobin; hence, argon laser tissue penetration is greater than that of ultraviolet (excimer) or far-infrared (CO_2) laser light.

Experimental studies. Beginning in 1980, a number of investigators showed that argon as well as Nd:YAG and CO_2 laser energy could be applied in vitro to vaporized post-mortem atherosclerotic specimens [7,8,10,11]. As expected, the magnitude of tissue vaporization was dependent on the amount of energy delivered (power [W] × pulse duration [s]). Histology reveals a characteristic "wedge"-shaped incision with a secondary zone of thermal injury. Additional in vitro studies using gas chromatography and mass spectrometry identified hydrogen, carbon monoxide, water vapors, and light hydrocarbon fragments as the byproducts formed in the gas phase after laser angioplasty. Absorption spectroscopy of the liquid media detected absorption in the ultraviolet region typical of protein fragments [12]. Thus, the concern for embolization of laser particulate material did not appear to be a significant risk.

However, it was not until successful in vivo transluminal laser angioplasty was reported using flexible argon laser fiberoptics in acutely thrombosed animal arteries [9] that real interest in laser angioplasty developed. In these early studies in experimental animals, a high incidence of vessel perforation was noted when the argon laser energy was emitted from bare fiberoptics positioned with fluoroscopic guidance alone [16,17].

Histologic studies after application of argon laser energy to normal and diseased vessels [2,3] revealed that typical laser craters could be created as had been observed in prior in vitro studies. In one study, in normal canine and atherosclerotic monkey aorta and large ileofemoral arteries, these laser-treated areas were covered with a layer of coagulated elements with only a few adherent platelets seen on scanning electron microscopy [13]. A healing response was noted in the first week after laser delivery, which consisted of a low-grade cellular infiltrate and reendothelialization. Most laser-treated segments were completely reendothelialized by 30–60 days, and no new dissection, occlusion thrombosis, or aneurysm formation was seen in this study in large peripheral arteries. In contrast, in smaller atherosclerotic rabbit iliac arteries [2], platelet and red cell thrombus formation was commonly seen after direct argon laser irradiation. Thus, vessel size and relative blood flow appear to play a role in the biological response to laser angioplasty.

Clinical studies in peripheral vessels. As in balloon angioplasty, in order to investigate the safety and efficacy of laser recanalization, this procedure was attempted in peripheral vessels first before considering coronary application. During this early phase of laser angioplasty investigation, several clinical trials were initiated with bare argon laser fiberoptics [5,6]. In these studies, a variety of laser powers and pulse durations were used to treat total or subtotal femoropopliteal occlusions prior to balloon angioplasty using a variety of laser approaches (antegrade or retrograde laser delivery). Lumen improvement on angiography was noted only in about 1/2 to 2/3 of patients after delivery of laser energy. Furthermore, despite the fact that the laser fiberoptics were positioned coaxially in the center of the arterial lumen inside angiographic or balloon catheters and the laser fiberoptics were withdrawn through previously recanalized lesions in the majority of cases, there still was a 15–20% incidence of vessel perforation.

Angioscopy has been proposed as one technique to aid laser angioplasty; however, in one study with direct angioscopic visualization of peripheral vascular lesions, there was actually a higher incidence of vessel perforation of approximately 50% [14] compared with the two previous studies [5,6] in which a fluoroscopic approach was used. Although angioscopy has not been useful during the performance of laser angioplasty, it may be better suited to evaluate intraluminal details of the angioplasty results if the technique can be perfected. Thus, the key limitations in these early clinical trials in peripheral vessels was the difficulty of controlling the narrow laser beam as it exited from the fiberoptic.

Intraoperative coronary laser recanalization. The feasibility of applying argon laser energy to human coronary arteries was first demonstrated intraoperatively during coronary artery bypass surgery [15]. In this initial report, laser recanalization was successful in three of five patients with one mechanical perforation; however, due in part to the influence of competitive flow from concurrent bypass surgery, no long-term patency greater than 3 months was present on follow-up angiography. Therefore, in addition to vessel perforation, laser recanalization with small 85 μm

diameter core fiberoptics created channels that were too small to maintain long-term patency.

Thus, modification of the laser delivery system was clearly needed to improve upon these results with argon fiberoptics. The first, but certainly not the last, argon laser fiberoptic to show promise in preliminary animal and clinical trials by demonstrating a high incidence of successful laser recanalization with a low incidence of vessel wall perforation is a laser-heated metallic-capped fiberoptic device (Laserprobe-PLR™, Trimedyne, Inc., Santa Ana, CA).

Nd:YAG Lasers

Laser properties. While the above argon laser angioplasty systems were being investigated, delivery systems were also being developed for the neodymium yttrium aluminium garnet (Nd:YAG) laser. Again, the availability and transmissibility down flexible fiberoptics were probably more instrumental in the early cardiovascular development of the Nd:YAG laser than were any particular laser property or laser-tissue interaction. As opposed to the above argon laser, which has gas as its laser medium, the Nd:YAG laser has a solid-state laser rod as its active media. The Nd:YAG laser emits near-infrared radiation at a wavelength of 1,060 nm (Table 1–1). This laser is quite versatile in that it can either operate from the CW mode with a high-average power up to 100 W or be pulsed through a technique called "Q-switching" to release intense high-peak-power pulses in the range of 10 ns through an optical feed-back mechanism. These high-power Q-switched pulses can be used to convert a substantial fraction of the 1,060 nm infrared radiation into visible green light at 532 nm or for additional conversion to 352 nm and 266 nm ultraviolet wavelengths. The infrared wavelengths of the Nd:YAG laser are absorbed less by atherosclerotic tissue than is the argon light; therefore, deeper penetration, more scattering, and more heat generation results with this laser. This property has made the Nd:YAG laser very effective for coagulation and tissue necrosis in other areas of medicine.

Experimental and clinical studies with bare Nd:YAG fiberoptics. As with the argon laser, initial in vitro and in vivo studies of Nd:YAG laser angioplasty used flexible silica fiberoptics positioned inside balloon catheters in order to maintain a central coaxial position and decrease the risk of vessel perforation [16,17]. In contrast to the prior studies with argon laser fiberoptics, a diluted blood perfusion of 3 mg/ dl hemoglobin concentration was used with the Nd:YAG laser system and found to be optimal for laser vaporization in the atherosclerotic lesion. Of note, too rapid an infusion of saline cooled the tissue and prevented thermal injury, whereas a slow rate of perfusion permitted blood to absorb the laser radiation and inhibit transfer of laser energy to the plaque.

Clinically, this Nd:YAG laser system was successful in recanalizing 12 femoropopliteal occlusions without perforation, but only narrow recanalized channels were obtained that required subsequent balloon dilation [17]. Histologic data obtained 2–4 weeks postprocedure in two patients revealed a rim of carbonization along the lumen, thermal injury, vacuolization of the intima, and no medial or elastic tissue disruption [18]. Interestingly, no evidence of thrombus formation was noted on histology after this CW laser delivery.

Modified Nd:YAG fiberoptic tips. Since the small (200 nm core diameter) fiberoptics used in the above studies created only small recanalized channels, attempts were made to modify the tips of these fiberoptics with lenses and sapphire contact probes in order to improve the efficacy as well as the safety of Nd:YAG laser angioplasty. In an in vitro study on human cadaver atherosclerotic arteries, a round 2.2 nm diameter sapphire contact probe was reported to be more effective than was a 1 mm diameter lensed fiberoptic [18]. In the first clinical experience with this Nd:YAG sapphire contact probe [19], successful laser recanalization to diameters of 2 mm or greater was reported in seven of eight attempts, with clinical improvement in at least five patients and one laser perforation.

As this Nd:YAG laser sapphire probe represents a rounded tip that requires tissue contact for effective vaporization, it probably has a mechanism of action that is very similar to the argon laser-heated metal probe. In addition, the metal probe has recently been used and approved by the FDA for use coupled to a Nd:YAG laser. If laser recanalization with larger, 3.5–5 mm diameter tips is desired in order to alleviate the need for subsequent balloon angioplasty, the more powerful Nd:YAG laser generator will probably be used rather than the argon laser generator. In the future, the clinical superiority of one system over the other one will depend more on various aspects of the catheter delivery system (i.e., flexibility, axial strength, and ability to pass over guidewires or "trackability").

PATHOPHYSIOLOGICAL MECHANISMS OF "CONTACT" LASER DEVICES

Laser Vaporization and Thermal Compression

Although there is a great deal of in vitro data that a variety of lasers can be used to vaporize atherosclerotic lesions, clinical angiography alone is unable to determine to what extent laser recanalization is true laser vaporization. The cardiovascular applications of lasers may actually involve several different pathophysiological mechanisms (Table 1–1). For example, in one previously mentioned study with the argon laser-heated metal probe [20], it was noted that increased pressure applied to the probe enhanced tissue ablation. It was postulated on the basis of histologic observations that *compression* of residual cellular and tissue components results in a decrease in the vacuolated cellular space. Thus, laser vaporization and thermal compression appear to be two important mechanisms of this "contact" laser approach to atherosclerotic lesions. Recent experimental studies suggest that the sapphire tips may have a similar mechanism of action [18]. Additional experimental studies are necessary to elucidate what proportion of laser recanalization is true laser vaporization of atherosclerotic mass and how much is mechanical enlargement of the lumen.

CONCLUSIONS

This has been a very brief overview of basic laser fundamentals and the early clinical experience with bare laser fiberoptics. For a more detailed discussion of laser physics, laser-tissue interactions, and other laser delivery systems, I would suggest an excellent review entitled *Lasers in Cardiovascular Disease,* which is edited by Drs. Rodney White and Warren Grundfest [21].

The present volume will deal entirely with clinical laser angioplasty including discussion of various approaches to the patient with peripheral arterial disease as well as individual techniques that have been used in this rapidly developing field. As this is a relatively new field and only one laser system has been approved by the FDA for use in peripheral arteries, the majority of the discussions will relate the use of one company's laser device (Laserprobe-PLR, Trimedyne, Inc., Santa Ana, CA). However, as new devices develop and results are presented, it is interesting to note the similarity of laser angioplasty techniques and approaches. Thus, the remainder of this volume should provide a useful "how-to" handbook of clinical laser angioplasty in its early stages.

REFERENCES

1. Sanborn TA, Faxon DP, Haudenschild CC, Gottsman SB, Ryan TJ: The mechanism of transluminal angioplasty; Evidence for formation of aneurysms in experimental atherosclerosis. Circulation 68:1136, 1983.

2. Sanborn TA, Faxon DP, Haudenschild CC, Ryan TJ: Experimental angioplasty: Circumferential distribution of

laser thermal energy with a laser probe. J Am Coll Cardiol 5:934, 1985.

3. Abela GS, Normann SJ, Cohen DM, Franzini D, Feldman RL, Crea F, Fenech A, Pepine CH, Conti CR: Laser recanalization of occluded atherosclerotic arteries in vivo and in vitro. Circulation 71:403, 1985.

4. Choy DSF, Stertzer SH, Myler RK, Marco J, Forunial G: Human coronary laser recanalization. Clin Cardiol 7:377, 1984.

5. Ginsburg R, Wexler L, Mitchell RS, Profitt D: Percutaneous transluminal laser angioplasty for treatment of peripheral vascular disease. Clinical experience with 16 patients. Radiology 156:619, 1985.

6. Cumberland DC, Taylor DI, Procter AE: Laser-assisted percutaneous angioplasty: Initial clinical experience in peripheral arteries. Clin Radiol 37:423, 1986.

7. Marcruz R, Martins JRM, Turpinanba AS, Lopes EA, Vargas H, Penaaf AE, Carvalaho VB, Armelin E, Decourt LV: Possibilidades terapeuticas do raio laser em ateromas (in Portuguese). Arq Bras Cardiol 34:9, 1980.

8. Lee G, Ikeda RM, Kozina J, Mason DT: Laser disolution of coronary atherosclerotic obstruction. Am Heart J 102:1074, 1981.

9. Choy DSJ, Stertzer S, Rotterdam HZ, Sharrock N, Kaminow IP: Transluminal laser catheter angioplasty. Am J Cardiol 50:1206, 1982.

10. Choy DSJ, Stertzer SH, Rotterdam HZ, Bruno MS: Laser coronary angioplasty: Experience with 9 cadaver hearts. Am J Cardiol 50:1209, 1982.

11. Abela GS, Normann S, Cohen D, Feldman RL, Geiser EA, Conti CR: Effects of carbon dioxide, Nd:YAG, and argon laser radiation on coronary atheromatous plaque. Am J Cardiol 60:1199, 1982.

12. Isner JM, Clarke RH, Donaldson RF, Aharon A: Identification of photoproducts liberated by in vitro argon laser irradiation of atherosclerotic plaque, calcified cardiac valves, and myocardium. Am J Cardiol 55:1192, 1985.

13. Abela GS, Crea F, Seeger JM, Franzini D, Fenech A, Normann S, Feldman RL, pepine CJ, Conti R: The healing process in normal canine arteries and in atherosclerotic monkey arteries after transluminal laser irradiation. Am J Cardiol 56:983, 1985.

14. Abela GS, Seeger JM, Barbieri E, Franzini D, Fenech A, Pepine CJ, Conti CR: Laser angioplasty with angioscopic guidance in humans. J Am Coll Cardiol 8:184, 1986.

15. Choy DSF, Stertzer SH, Myler RK, Marco J, Forunial G: Human coronary laser recanalization. Clin Cardiol 7:377, 1984.

16. Geschwind HJ, Boussignac G, Teisseire B, Benhaiem N, Bittoun R, Laurent D: Conditions for effective Nd-YAG laser angioplasty. Br Heart J 52:484, 1984.

17. Geschwind H, Fabre M, Chaitman BR, Lefebvre-Villardebo M, Ladouch A, Boussignac G, Blair JD, Kennedy HL: Histopathology after Nd-YAG laser percutaneous transluminal angioplasty of peripheral arteries. J Am Coll Cardiol 8:1089, 1986.

18. Geschwind HJ, Kern MJ, Vandormael MG, Blair JD, Deligonul U, Kennedy HL: Efficiency and safety of optically modified fiber tips for laser angioplasty. J Am Coll Cardiol 10:655, 1987.

19. Fourrier JL, Brunetaud JM, Prat A, Marache P, Lablanche JM, Bertrand ME: Percutaneous laser angioplasty with sapphire tip. Lancet I:105, 1987.

20. Welch AJ, Bradley AB, Torres JH, Motamedi M, Ghidori JJ, Pearse JA, Hussein H, O'Rourke RA: Laser probe ablation of normal and atherosclerotic human aortic in vitro: A first thermographic and histologic analysis. Circulation 76:1353–1563, 1987.

21. White RA, Grundfest WS: Lasers in Cardiovascular Disease. Chicago: Year Book Medical Publishers, Inc., 1987.

2. Noninvasive Vascular Laboratory Evaluation: Applications for Laser Angioplasty

Jonathan L. Halperin, M.D.

INTRODUCTION

The modern clinical vascular noninvasive laboratory is subject to misconceptions that predispose to misuse. Among these are that laboratory findings can establish the indications for laser angioplasty; however, test results serve this purpose no better than they determine when vascular reconstructive surgery—or any other intervention—is appropriate. Such clinical decisions are best made on the basis of symptoms and the physical appearance of involved tissues. The laboratory provides information, however, which may be helpful in judging the severity of ischemia, the contribution of obstructive arterial factors to symptoms, and the absolute and relative hemodynamic significance of lesions at various points along the course of the arterial circulation. Currently available noninvasive technology furnishes an objective perspective along anatomic and functional as well as hemodynamic lines, and this has become virtually essential to clinical practice [1].

Even before there was catheter angioplasty, there was a role for vascular laboratory measurements as a qualitative and quantitative guide during clinical follow-up of medically or surgically treated patients. When balloon dilatation of arterial stenoses became the mainstay of interventional angiography, available noninvasive technology did not permit reliable distinction of occlusive from nonocclusive arterial lesions. Methods of imaging the morphology of arterial obstructions appeared coincidentally with the successful application of laser angioplasty to occluded arterial segments. As the science of thermal angioplasty has evolved through sequential stages of feasibility testing, early clinical development, and demonstration of practical utility, the problem of case selection for angioplasty or surgery still extends beyond whatever angiographic features of disease might make the patient an anatomic candidate for any given means of restoring circulation. When the state of the patient's general health is poor, or claudication

occurs without impairment of perfusion at rest, medical wisdom may mitigate against a surgical approach. Objective laboratory data are widely employed to classify cases of chronic lower extremity ischemia in standardized terms of severity (Table 2–1). Beyond this, the measurements add objectivity to preinterventional assessment and provide a benchmark for estimation of the hemodynamic outcome. Test results are senseless when taken out of clinical context, but provide an additional dimension along which clinical insight can be extended.

DIAGNOSIS OF ARTERIAL OBSTRUCTIVE DISEASE

Arterial obstructive disease of the lower extremities is currently the main target of angioplasty, though experience is growing in the upper extremity arteries and in vessels other than those of the limbs. The principal lesions are overwhelmingly atherosclerotic, but obstructions are sometimes encountered that are caused by other disease entities, among them giant cell arteritis, fibromuscular dysplasia, thromboangiitis obliterans, and vascular tumors.

Evaluation of the patient with arteriosclerosis obliterans begins in the office or at the bedside with identification of the cardinal symptoms: intermittent claudication, ischemic rest pain, or necrotic gangrene. Physical examination is directed toward differential diagnosis—considering, for example, dynamic compression by extravascular structures, vasospasm, neurogenic pseudoclaudication, embolic phenomena, and other causes of discomfort, disability, or tissue destruction—and toward estimation of the location and severity of arterial pathology. Examination should focus on the signs of acute tissue ischemia (petechiae, regional edema, tenderness, ulceration, and gangrene), as well as the trophic signs of chronic ischemia (subcutaneous atrophy, brittle toenails, hair loss, pallor, coolness, or dependent rubor), sympathetic denervation (absence of regional sweating and disorganization of the hair pattern due to piloerector involvement), and signs of sensorimotor neuropathy (impaired perception of vibration and fine touch and diminished deep tendon reflexes). Pal-

Laser Angioplasty, pages 7–14
© 1989 Alan R. Liss, Inc.

TABLE 2–1. Clinical Categories of Chronic Limb Ischemia

Grade	Category	Clinical description	Objective criteria
0	0	Asymptomatic—no hemodynamically significant occlusive disease	Normal treadmill/stress test
I	1	Mild claudication	Completes treadmill exercise[a]; AP after exercise, 25–50 mm Hg less than BP
	2	Moderate claudication	Between categories 1 and 3
	3	Severe claudication	Cannot complete treadmill test; AP after exercise < 50 mm Hg
II	4	Ischemic rest pain	Resting AP < 40 mm Hg, flat or barely pulsatile ankle or metatarsal PVR; TP < 30 mm Hg
III	5	Minor tissue loss nonhealing ulcer, focal gangrene with diffuse pedal ischemia	Resting AP < 60 mm Hg, ankle or metatarsal PVR flat or barely pulsatile; TP < 40 mm Hg
	6	Major tissue loss extending above TM level, functional foot no longer salvageable	Same as category 5

Data prepared by the ad-hoc committee on reporting standards, Society for Vascular Surgery/North American Chapter, International Society for Cardiovascular Surgery [2].
[a]Five minutes at 2 mph on a 12% incline.
Abbreviations: AP = ankle pressure; BP = brachial pressure; PVR = pulse-volume recording; TP = toe pressure; TM = transmetatarsal.

pation of the femoral, popliteal, posterior tibial, and dorsalis pedis pulses is performed in conjunction with auscultation of the abdomen and groins for arterial bruits. These regional systolic murmurs denote the presence of turbulent flow and imply arterial disease, but whether the sonic characteristics of bruits reflect the severity of obstruction remains controversial [3]. Cutaneous perfusion pressure may be estimated by assessing the color and temperature of the feet during elevation above the level of the heart, at rest, and following gastrocnemius muscle exercise. Standardized observations correlate remarkably closely with objective measurements of distal pressure made in the laboratory [4]. Next, collateral perfusion can be gauged upon dependency, by timing the hyperemic return of pink color to the skin of the foot, and the development of venous refilling (unless the latter is accelerated by concomitant venous insufficiency), which provide a crude but dependable index of flow in physiologic terms, along the dimensions of blood volume, tissue mass, and time.

DOPPLER SPHYGMOMANOMETRY

The clinical examination is readily supplemented by Doppler velocity stethoscopy and sphygmomanometry, which have become standard parts of the initial examination of the vascular disease patient at the bedside. The Doppler ultrasound stethoscope is employed in conjunction with a standard brachial-sized sphygmomanometric cuff for determination of the ankle:arm systolic blood pressure index. The cuff is placed around the ankle and the Doppler stethoscope is used to detect pulsatile arterial blood flow over the dorsalis pedis or posterior tibial arteries, or beneath the plantar arterial arch. The cuff is then inflated to the point at which arterial pulsations become obliterated; this is registered as the systolic arterial pressure at the level of cuff application (not at the level of flow detection with the Doppler probe). Here, the Doppler device serves principally as a flow detector; its use is largely obviated if arterial pulses are palpable or if sounds of Korotkoff can be identified by auscultation with the conventional stethoscope.

Normally, systolic arterial pressure at the ankle exceeds that obtained by the same method over the brachial artery, as both systolic pressure and pulse pressure tend to increase as the pulse wave propagates from the heart [5]. An ankle:arm systolic pressure ratio (tibial:brachial index) less than unity at rest indicates hemodynamically significant arterial obstruction proximal to the leg cuff. With constant cuff position, finding major differences in readings as flow is detected at various points implies arterial obstructive disease distal to the popliteal trifurcation. Advanced, calcific atherosclerotic changes in vessels directly beneath the pneumatic cuff may resist compression, producing overestimation of regional perfusion pressure. This constitutes the major limitation of sphygmomanometry and may lead to falsely elevated tibial:brachial pressure indices. One must be particularly alert to this possibility in patients with diabetes mellitus, even when glucose intolerance is comparatively mild; patients with chronic renal failure are also prone to arterial calcification.

Just as arterial pulses may remain palpable distally in patients with severe proximal arterial obstructive lesions, so the systolic pressure and tibial:brachial index may appear within the normal range at rest. Analysis of recordings of Doppler analog signals has disclosed characteristic velocity waveform changes in the presence of hemodynamic obstruction depending on the location and severity of stenosis, and, with practice, these can be subjectively assessed with the Doppler stethoscope. Reliability is lost from one listener to the next, however, and the method is not regularly incorporated into clinical practice. The single most sensitive bedside test for hemodynamically significant arterial stenosis is a decline in the pressure index following exercise of the calf muscles, which usually remains below the baseline (resting) value for several minutes. Indeed, with the exception of cases of vascular noncompressibility, this stands as one of the simplest, most effective means of screening for hemodynamically significant arterial obstructive disease. Postexercise systolic pressure readings below 90 mm Hg are typical of patients with intermittent claudication, and values below 60 mm Hg are usually encountered in patients with ulcerative ischemia at rest.

SEGMENTAL PRESSURE MEASUREMENT

In order to localize one or more segmental arterial lesions, appropriately sized pneumatic cuffs are applied to various points on the limb to determine systolic pressure at several levels simultaneously. The principle is that obstruction must be proximal to the level at which pressure drops. In most laboratories, a pulse sensor is employed in conjunction with automatically inflatable segmental pressure cuffs for this purpose. Segmental pressure measurements are typically obtained in both lower extremities along with pulse-volume recordings, using cuffs with bladders 36 × 18 cm for the upper thighs (placed below the level of the groins) and lower thighs (positioned just above the knees) and 22 × 12 cm for the calves and ankles; smaller digital cuffs are used for more distal measurements. Pressure is determined at the site of the proximal occluding cuff when its pressure obliterates the pulse detected with the distal sensor. Data may be interpreted in terms of the pressure gradient between two adjacent sites in an extremity by comparing the values in opposite limbs or by calculation of the pressure ratio with reference to brachial systolic readings (Fig. 2–1). After resting values are obtained, the patient can exercise by walking on a treadmill, following which the cuffs are quickly reconnected to the inflation system and recorder.

In general, segmental pressure measurements made in this fashion are subject to the same limitations as

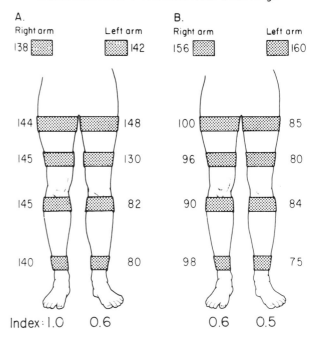

SEGMENTAL PRESSURES (mm Hg)

Fig. 2–1. Segmental limb systolic pressures and tibial:brachial indices. **A,** Left superficial femoral arterial obstructive disease. **B,** Bilateral aortoiliac obstructive disease.

Doppler sphygmomanometry at the ankle. In addition, it is important to recognize that thigh pressure measurements may underestimate pressure in the common femoral artery, falsely suggesting arterial obstruction at the aortoiliac level. In such cases, Doppler velocity waveforms obtained from the femoral artery at the groin appear normal. On the other hand, normal pressures at the level of the thigh cuff do not exclude significant stenosis in either the profunda femoris or superficial femoral arteries. In general, leg:arm systolic pressure indices over 0.85 occur in individuals without obstructive disease; values between 0.5 and 0.8 are typical at rest in patients with intermittent claudication, and values below 0.5 are frequently associated with ischemic rest pain, ulceration, and gangrene threatening the viability of the limb. Partly because of arterial rigidity, systolic ankle pressures may be high in patients with diabetes mellitus even when limb loss is threatened [6].

PULSE-VOLUME RECORDING

The quantitative segmental pneumatic plethysmograph is widely employed in conjunction with pressure measurements to monitor arterial wall motion indirectly, using sensor cuffs inflated to approximately 30–80 mm Hg to generate waveforms of optimum fidelity.

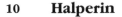

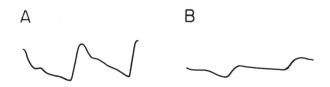

Fig. 2–2. Segmental pulse-volume recordings obtained with pneumatic cuff transducers. **A,** Left thigh tracing of a patient with claudication and obstructive disease of the popliteal artery. **B,** Left calf waveform taken simultaneously in the same patient.

The amplitude of the pulse-volume recording reflects local arterial pressure, vascular wall compliance, the number of arterial vessels beneath the cuff, and the severity of atherosclerotic disease. As pressure in a proximal occluding cuff is reduced below systolic level, pulse-wave amplitude increases in the monitoring cuff to a maximum as diastolic arterial pressure is reached beneath the occluding cuff. Results are generally within 10 mm Hg of direct intraarterial measurements, with systolic pressure slightly lower and diastolic pressure higher by the indirect technique.

The normal digital pulse is characterized by a sharp systolic upstroke, rises rapidly to a peak, and then drops off more slowly toward the baseline. The downslope is curved toward the baseline and usually contains a more or less prominent dicrotic notch and secondary wave about midway between the peak and the baseline. This dicrotic wave is apparently caused by the reflection of the arterial pulse from the periphery. The pulse recorded distal to an arterial obstruction differs in several ways: The general shape is more rounded and the anacrotic slope is reduced; the crest is delayed and the catacrotic limb descends more gradually; and the dicrotic (reflected diastolic) wave is lost (Fig. 2–2).

Segmental compression cuffs combined with the Doppler ultrasound device, photoplethysmograph, or other flow detector are subject to error related to arterial rigidity, but the pulse-volume recorder, using either pneumatic cuffs or mercury-in-Silastic strain gauges to reflect arterial wall motion, has the advantage of revealing distortions in pulse-wave contour even in patients with vascular calcification. The pulse waveforms appear depressed and altered even when arteries are noncompressible. The pulsatility index, representing the ratio of pulse amplitude to mean volume obtained by integration of the deflection, is abnormally low even when systolic pressure readings are falsely elevated. This principle underlies the use of aneroid oscillometry, which can provide a semiquantitative index of arterial pulse pressure at the bedside. Unfortunately, the fragility of the aneroid capsules employed in portable oscillometer equipment makes calibration errors common.

Serial analysis of digital pulse contours during fol-low-up of laser angioplasty patients allows comparison of various technical modifications if such factors as ambient temperature and sympathetic nervous system activity are considered. More importantly, the detailed recording of digital pulse waves may be of value is assessing sympathetic tone, contributing to decisions regarding sympathectomy or interpreting the pathophysiology of impaired wound healing in diabetic patients.

VENOUS-OCCLUSION PLETHYSMOGRAPHY

Venous-occlusion plethysmography using either volume-displacement or segmental strain-gauge apparatus has been in use longer than most methods currently employed in clinical vascular diagnostic laboratories, and the technique remains the standard for measurement of perfusion in a portion of a limb. Nevertheless, its major application is in physiologic studies of vasomotor activity, since isolated measurements of resting blood flow are not helpful in distinguishing normal limbs from those with significant obstructive lesions. Flow measurements become depressed at rest only when ischemia is fairly advanced and vasodilator reserve has been exhausted. Recovery of perfusion after exercise and postischemic reactive hyperemia approximate maximum vasodilatation and effectively differentiate normal from impaired circulation. The methodology is cumbersome and used mainly to assess collateral resistance and hemorheologic variables affecting treatment [7].

RADIONUCLIDE MAPPING

Microspheres amenable to radionuclide labeling are commercially available, and medical diagnostic use is based on the assumption that distribution of particulate material injected into the arterial circulation is identical to that of blood flowing to the capillary microcirculation. There are four specific requirements of practical importance in the application of this method for study of limb circulation: 1) biocompatibility, 2) prompt, uniform dispersion of the particles in arterial blood, 3) distribution at arterial branch points in proportion to blood flow, and 4) complete first-pass extraction at the level of the microcirculation.

The greatest material success at lower extremity perfusion imaging has been achieved with [99m]technicium-labeled microaggregated albumin. In patients with atheroclerosis studied at the time of translumbar aortography, blood flow distribution in the lower extremities was indistinguishable from that in normal individuals. During reactive hyperemia following relief of ischemia, however, variations in distribution of radioactive microspheres correlated with arteriographic findings and subjective symptoms in 83% of cases [8,9].

Similar applications have validated predictive value for spontaneous healing of ischemic ulcers [10]. In general, however, radioactive microsphere distribution techniques have not been clinically valuable, since peripheral arterial injection provides nonquantitative information about flow distribution. Radionuclide angiography using technetium-labeled autologous erythrocytes provides insufficient image quality for therapeutically directed assessment of atherosclerotic lesions, but is useful for study of arteriovenous anastomoses.

The local clearance of isotopes has proven simpler and provides reliable quantitative data related to regional blood flow. In this method, a small volume (0.02–0.05 ml) of a solution of radioactive tracer, typically xenon in saline, is injected locally into tissue such as tibialis or gastrocnemius muscle and the rate of disappearance is extrapolated to blood flow assuming a monoexponential function. At rest, results obtained in patients with arterial disease are often in the normal range and, again, hyperemic methods are recruited to enhance diagnostic value. The technique has the advantage of reproducibility, and one intriguing observation has been that exercise training of patients with claudication, although improving walking tolerance, does not increase the rate of xenon clearance from calf skeletal muscle [11]. The major limitation is that perfusion is gauged in a very small region of tissue, and local perfusion imbalance may drastically influence results; larger volumes of injectate, though, may induce direct changes in blood flow. [201]Thallium imaging of lower limb musculature at rest in comparison with exercise has also been of limited value in verifying areas of relative ischemia, but depends too heavily upon heterogeneity of perfusion to be of much practical benefit.

The future clearly promises more specific metabolically based isotope selection and positron emission tomography for assessment of vascular disease, but data are presently insufficient for comprehensive evaluation. A fruitful area in the years upcoming seems to be that of tracer-labeled lipoprotein imaging of atherosclerotic lesions or [111]indium-labeled platelet imaging to examine the immediate tissue injury induced during laser angioplasty [12–14].

ECHO-DOPPLER (DUPLEX) ULTRASOUND IMAGING

Duplex ultrasound scanning provides a direct, noninvasive test of both functional and anatomic characteristics of arterial obstructive lesions. The methodology combines B-mode ultrasound imaging and pulsed Doppler velocity analysis to examine arterial configuration and localized velocity information at sites of stenosis. The pulsed Doppler sample volume detector is guided by the ultrasound image to specific arterial locations. The angle of incidence of the Doppler beam with the vessel axis is measured and used to derive velocity information, which is recorded graphically as a function of time. The amplitude of the velocity signal is indicated by shades of gray, or with directional vectors when color flow imaging is available. Flow through a stenosis is accelerated, and turbulence related to the configuration of the obstruction is detected as spectral broadening of the band of particulate velocities, instead of the narrow band seen with normal laminar flow.

Application of this technique to lower extremity arteries was delayed by technical limitations involving transducer design. High-frequency apparatus proved satisfactory for relatively superficial arteries, but could not be used for deeper structures, which required lower transducer frequencies in the range of 2.5 MHz. Both the focal point of the flow detector and the sampling volume had to be adjustable to accommodate vessels of varying diameters lying at different depths and that, in the abdomen, varied with respiration. These capabilities now coexist with fast Fourier transformations of the velocity spectrum and microprocessor-based systems for calculation of actual blood cell velocities, allowing precise estimation of instantaneous pressure gradients and degrees of stenosis.

The ultrasound imaging procedure is performed with the patient supine and the lower extremities slightly rotated externally. The aorta is imaged in the midline just below the level of the xiphoid, using a 3 MHz transducer, and traced distally to the level of the iliac bifurcation; each iliac artery can be examined to the groin. The common, deep, and superficial femoral arteries are imaged in the adductor canal (Fig. 2–3). The patient is positioned prone for examination of the popliteal fossae, with the feet elevated about 30°. The origins of the tibial arteries can usually be identified, but detailed examination of the distal tibial-peroneal arteries is technically difficult. More superficial arteries are studied with 5.0- and 7.5 MHz transducers. Waveforms are recorded from each accessible arterial segment, and detailed analysis is performed for each area in which disturbed flow is detected.

Normal arterial vessels show a triphasic velocity signal. Rapid acceleration to peak systolic velocity occurs along a narrow frequency spectrum. End-systolic deceleration culminates in protodiastolic reversal of flow, the amplitude of which is inversely proportional to the dynamic peripheral resistance, including rheologic factors. Antegrade flow resumes in mid-diastole as a consequence of the *windkessel* recoil effect in the proximal

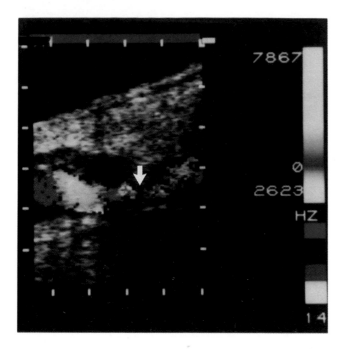

Fig. 2–3. Duplex color-coded Doppler ultrasound image of left femoral artery at the site of hemodynamically significant stenosis (arrow).

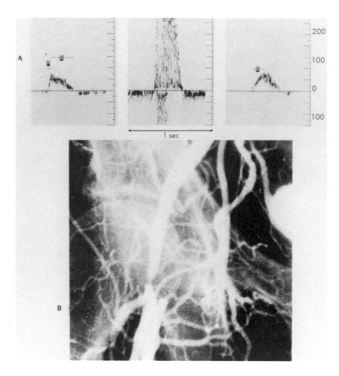

Fig. 2–4. **A,** Pulsed-Doppler velocity spectra obtained proximal to, at the site of, and distal to a stenotic lesion. **B,** Corresponding femoral arteriographic findings. Reproduced with permission of K.A. Jager, H.J. Richetts, and D.E. Strandness (Duplex scanning for the evaluation of lower limb arterial disease. In Bernstein EF (ed): Noninvasive Diagnostic Techniques in Vascular Disease, 3rd Ed. St. Louis: The C.V. Mosby Company, 1985).

aorta. Peak systolic velocities diminish with advancing age, but are not significantly different in males than in females, despite smaller arterial diameters in women.

In mild arterial stenosis, involving less than about 20% narrowing of the luminal diameter, spectral broadening of the Doppler velocity signal is detected, but peak velocity and the triphasic waveform remain within the normal range. Peak systolic velocity accelerates 30–100% (with respect to a proximal, adjacent arterial segment) when there is about 50% stenosis, and spectral broadening is present, but normal velocity patterns are detected proximal and distal to the lesion. Beyond this degree of stenosis, the velocity waveform becomes monophasic as the reversal of protodiastolic flow ceases; peak systolic velocity is more than double that in the immediately proximal portion of the artery. At the site of arterial stenosis, velocity is accelerated and spectral broadening is marked. Distal to the stenosis, flow usually remains monophasic, but peak velocity is reduced (Fig. 2–4). Total occlusion is characterized by absence of flow in the imaged vessel and markedly distorted proximal and distal velocity waveforms. When multiple levels of stenosis are present, relative increases in velocity still occur across each lesion, but the magnitude of the changes decreases as proximal lesions become more severe. In such cases, the gradients across distal lesions may be estimated less accurately.

Initial clinical studies comparing duplex ultrasound scanning with angiography found a sensitivity of 77%,

specificity of 98%, positive predictive value of 94%, and negative predictive value of 92% for lesions reducing arterial diameter more than 50% [15]. It is intriguing that these results were not affected much by multisegmental disease. The overall concordance (k = 0.69) compares favorably with interobserver differences in angiographic interpretation of severity of stenoses. Experience has been particularly favorable for the iliac and superficial femoral arteries, but errors are more frequent in the profunda femoral artery and it is difficult to obtain an adequate examination below the trifurcation of the popliteal artery.

Duplex scanning is effective as a means of localizing and classifying peripheral arterial stenoses. It has particular advantages over other noninvasive methods for the evaluation of aortoiliac disease. Stenoses potentially amenable to angioplasty can be identified in patients who represent less than optimal candidates for angiography. No other noninvasive method is as useful for distinguishing critical stenosis from occlusion, which may have direct bearing on the angioplasty technique selected. Duplex scanning is more sensitive and specific than are segmental blood pressure measurements for detection of restenosis, which can be detected by the ultrasound method even before pressure drops [16–17].

TISSUE CHARACTERIZATION

More sophisticated ultrasound tissue characterization techniques are presently under development that may allow precise descriptions of the atherosclerotic lesions themselves as fibrotic, lipoid, thrombotic, hyperplastic, calcific, etc. and lead to more rational understanding of the impact of laser energy upon this diversity of tissue types. While platelet accumulation, lipid deposition, fibrosis, and calcification cannot be reliably assessed by conventional sonographic means, the interactions of ultrasound with tissue and blood have yielded encouraging data in observations of both the heart and blood vessels. Unprocessed ultrasonic backscatter signals have been acquired even from conventional imaging systems, digitized, corrected for physical and system factors, and analyzed for tissue signature using a variety of frequency- and time-domain methods. In excised aortic and iliac arterial segments, at least four histological categories have been acoustically differentiated (normal, fatty, fibrous, and calcific) [18–24] and ultrasound reflectance changes related to blood coagulation, temperature, and flow velocity have been documented both in vitro and in vivo [25–29].

In the future, we may look to the ultrasound probe for initial evaluation of patients considering angioplasty, evaluate morphologic candidacy of arterial lesions, and predict rates of immediate recanalization and long-term success; the same method could be employed for postinterventional observations. This technology will doubtless compete, however, with advances in the fields of positron emission tomography of the atherosclerotic lesions and magnetic resonance imaging.

FUTURE PERSPECTIVE

We may anticipate that, in the future, noninvasive tests will select potential candidates for angioplasty prior to or without the need for contrast angiography. In this respect, the vascular laboratory holds the promise of identifying patients with conditions suitable for angioplasty so that the ticket to clinical decision making will no longer carry the cost of an invasive procedure without direct therapeutic potential. Beyond the horizon, the vascular noninvasive laboratory offers not only to enhance the clinical and angiographic principles upon which standards of diagnosis and the evaluation of treatment are based, but also to advance our understanding of the mechanisms of clinical success and failure.

REFERENCES

1. Nicolaides AN: The preoperative selection of patients—What must the surgeon know? In Bernstein EF (ed): Noninvasive Diagnostic Techniques in Vascular Disease, 2nd Ed. St. Louis: CV Mosby, 1982:311–316.

2. Rutherford RB, Flanigan DP, Gupta SK, Johnston KW, Karmody A, Wittemore AD, Baker JD, Ernst CB: Suggested standards for reports dealing with lower extremity ischemia. J Vasc Surg 4:80–94, 1986.

3. Lees RS, Miller A, Kistler JP: Quantitative carotid phonoangiography. In Nicolaides A, Yao J (eds): The Investigation of Vascular Disorders. Edinburgh: Churchill Livingstone, 1981.

4. Lorentsen E: The plantar ischemia test (contribution to the discussion about local blood pressure measurements in patients with peripheral arterial insufficiency). Scand J Clin Lab Invest (Suppl 128) 31:149–150, 1973.

5. Taylor MG: Wave travel in arteries and the design of the cardiovascular system. In Attinger EO (ed): Pulsatile Blood Flow. New York: McGraw-Hill, 1964.

6. Bernstein EF: How does a vascular laboratory influence management of arterial disease? In Greenhalgh RM, Jamieson CW, Nicolaides AN (eds): Vascular Surgery: Issues in Current Practice. London: Grune & Stratton, 1986:101–105.

7. Halperin JL, Rothlauf EB, Stern A: Potential adverse effect of pentoxifylline on limb hemodynamics in patients with intermittent claudication. J Am Coll Cardiol 7:177A, 1986.

8. Siegel ME, Giargiana FA Jr., Rhodes BA, White I, Wagner HN: Effect of reactive hyperemia on the distribution of radioactive microspheres in patients with peripheral vascular disease. AJR 118:814–819, 1973.

9. Siegel ME, Giargiana FA Jr., White RI Jr., Friedman H, Wagner H: Peripheral vascular perfusion scanning: Correlation with the arteriogram and clinical assessment in the patient with peripheral vascular disease. AJR 125:628–633, 1975.

10. Siegel ME, Giargiana FA Jr., Rhodes BA, Williams GM, Wagner HN: Perfusion of ischemic ulcers of the extremity: A prognostic indicator of healing. Arch Surg 110:265–268, 1976.

11. Lassen NA, Holstein P: Use of radioisotopes in assessment of distal blood flow and distal blood pressure in arterial insufficiency. Surg Clin North Am 54:39–55, 1974.

12. Lam JYT, Chesebro JH, Steele PM, Deulangee MK, Badimon L, Fuster V, Byrne JM, Lamb HB, Wendland BI: Deep arterial injury during experimental angioplasty: Relation to a positive [111]indium-labeled platelet scintigram, quantitative platelet deposition and mural thrombosis. J Am Coll Cardiol 8:1380–1386, 1986.

13. Pope CF, Ezekowitz MD, Smith EO, Rapoport S, Glickman M, Sostman HD, Zaret B: Detection of platelet

deposition at the site of peripheral ballon angioplasty using [111]indium platelet scintigraphy. Am J Cardiol 55:495–497, 1985.

14. Cunningham DA, Kumar B, Siegel BA, Gilula LA, Totty WG, Welen MJ: Aspirin inhibition of platelet deposition at angioplasty sites: demonstration by platelet scintigraphy. Radiology 151:487–490, 1984.

15. Samson RH, Sprayregan S, Veith FJ, Gupta SK, Ascer E, Scher LA: Inadequacy of the noninvasive hemodynamic evaluation of percutaneous transluminal angioplasty. Am J Surg 147:212–215, 1984.

16. Gunn IG, Cowie TN, Forrest H, Quin RO, Sheldon C, Vallance R: Haemodynamic assessment following iliac dilatation. Br J Surg 68:858–860, 1981.

17. Kohler TR, Strandness DE: Duplex scanning of peripheral arteries: Practical application. In Bergan JJ, Yao JST (eds): Arterial Surgery: New Diagnostic and Operative Techniques. Orlando, FL: Grune & Stratton, 1988:437–446.

18. Barzilai B, Saffitz JE, Miller JG, Sobel BE: Quantitative ultrasonic characterization of the nature of atherosclerotic plaques in human aorta. Circ Res 60:459–463, 1987.

19. Miller JG, Perez JE, Sobel BE: Ultrasonic characterization of myocardium. Prog Cardiovasc Dis 110:28–85, 1985.

20. Landini L, Sarnelli R, Picano E, Salvador M: Evaluation of frequency dependence of backscatter coefficient in normal and atherosclerotic aortic walls. Ultrasound Med Biol 12:397–401, 1986.

21. Picano E, Landini L, Lattanzi F, Mazzarisi A, Sarnelli R, Distante A, Benassi A, L'Abbate A: The use of frequency histograms of ultrasonic backscatter amplitudes for detection of atherosclerosis in vitro. Circulation 74:1093–1098, 1986.

22. Picano E, Landini L, Distante A, Sarnelli R, Benassi A, L'Abbate A: Different degrees of atherosclerosis detected by backscatter ultrasound: An in vitro study on fixed human aortic walls. J Clin Ultrasound 2:375–379, 1983.

23. Wolverson MK, Heiberg E, Sundaram M, Tantanasirviangse S, Shields JB: Carotid atherosclerosis: High resolution real-time sonography correlated with angiography. AJR 140:355–361, 1983.

24. Bronez MA, Shung KK, Heidary H, Hurwitz D: Measurement of ultrasound velocity in tissues utilizing a microprocessor-based system. IEEE Trans Biomed Eng 32:723–726, 1985.

25. Shung KK, Siulgelmann RA, Reid JM: Scattering of ultrasound by blood. IEEE Trans Biomed Eng 23:460–467, 1977.

26. Shung KK, Fei DY, Ballard JO: Further studies on ultrasonic properties of blood clots. J Clin Ultrasound 14:269–275, 1986.

27. Shung KK, Fei DY, Yuan YW, Reeves WC: Ultrasonic characterization of blood during coagulation. J Clin Ultrasound 12:147–153, 1984.

28. Green SE, Joynt LF, Fitzgerald PJ, Rubenson DS, Popp RL: In vivo ultrasonic tissue characterization of human intracardiac masses. Am J Cardiol 51:231–236, 1983.

29. Sigel B, Machi J, Beitler JC, Justin JR, Coelho JCU: Variable ultrasound echogenicity in flowing blood. Science 218:1321–1323, 1982.

3. Peripheral Angioplasty Techniques

Alan J. Greenfield, M.D.

INTRODUCTION

Since its introduction by Dotter and Judkins in 1964 [1], percutaneous transluminal angioplasty (PTA) has undergone continuous technical development, as well as revolutionary changes, the most significant of which was the development of the balloon catheter by Andreas Gruntzig [2]. With the development of atheroablative techniques, we are entering a new stage in the development of percutaneous atherosurgery. The safe use of these new modalities is founded on facility with proven techniques for safe access to the peripheral vessels. In addition, many of the newer techniques can be used only as adjuncts to conventional balloon angioplasty and actually are means to broaden the scope of patients amenable to treatment by classic percutaneous techniques. As a result, the use of lasers for recanalization of occluded vessels demands an excellent understanding of traditional angioplasty.

PATIENT SELECTION

Appropriate selection of patients for angioplasty is discussed in other chapters (see chaps. 2, 5–10), and most of the important criteria are covered at length. In addition to the usual criteria that are considered in accepting patients for treatment of limb ischemia (severity of ischemia and type and location of lesion), certain patient factors that affect the technical outcome of the procedure must be considered when choosing candidates for laser angioplasty.

Patient habitus must be considered when infrainguinal angioplasty is required. Antegrade puncture becomes considerably more challenging when a large pannus must be dealt with, because catheter manipulation is more difficult, especially when an introduction sheath is required, and postprocedure hemostasis is harder to achieve. The relationship of the profunda femoris bifurcation to the inguinal ligament must be carefully examined, since, ideally, puncture is best made in the common femoral artery. Superficial fem-

oral artery puncture can be employed occasionally, but is considered more risky. Large patients with high femoral bifurcations may best be treated via surgical exposure of the common femoral artery, with puncture of the exposed vessel under direct vision. An additional advantage of this approach is that much better hemostasis is achieved. However, there is more morbidity and a longer recovery period using this approach. The current generation of lasers does not support the contralateral over-the-bifurcation approach. An additional issue to be considered is the presence of previous surgical reconstruction, since prosthetic grafts at the puncture sites make catheter manipulation more difficult. Again, surgical exposure can be useful in this instance.

The patient's underlying disease must be considered, with the most important factor being renal function. Careful assessment must be made of the probable difficulty of the procedure, with consequent increase in contrast requirement. Since, even in the best of hands, patients may require urgent surgical intervention, the patient should be evaluated as a possible surgical candidate and his/her health status maximized. Patients without threatened limbs, who are otherwise poor surgical risks, must be carefully apprised of the risks involved in surgical correction of a technical misadventure.

PATIENT PREPARATION

General preparation for PTA is similar to that for diagnostic arteriography. This includes evaluation of renal function and clotting studies. Noninvasive vascular evaluation is obtained to provide a baseline against which to evaluate results. The diagnostic arteriogram should be repeated if it was performed more than 2 weeks prior to the angioplasty, since a considerable extension of involvement can occur with little or no clinical deterioration.

Most radiologists performing angioplasty routinely start ASA treatment 24 h prior to the procedure; while experimental evidence strongly supports its use [3], no formal study of its usefulness in peripheral angioplasty has been performed. In order to reduce renal toxicity from contrast, the patient should be well hy-

Laser Angioplasty, pages 15–20
© 1989 Alan R. Liss, Inc.

drated, both with routine IV therapy prior to the procedure and by allowing the patient liquids on the day of the procedure.

TECHNICAL ISSUES IN PERFORMING ANGIOPLASTY

Percutaneous Techniques for the Distal Aorta and Iliac Vessels

While laser angioplasty at present seems to have a more limited role in the management of aortoiliac atherosclerosis, recent work suggests that occlusive disease of the iliac system may become a legitimate target [4]. In order to avoid balloon angioplasty, the most successful reported technique requires surgical exposure to introduce large-diameter probes. Unfortunately, this requirement eliminates one of the benefits of a percutaneous technique.

Access. Iliac angioplasty is usually performed via retrograde puncture of the ipsilateral common femoral artery. Occasionally, when the anatomy of the lesion to be treated makes it difficult to traverse the lesion safely from a retrograde approach, the contralateral femoral artery can be chosen, and antegrade traversal of the diseased arterial segment accomplished "around the horn." This is often considerably more difficult than the antegrade approach because of severe involvement of the aortic bifurcation. Newer laser-probe catheters that will follow a wire may make this alternate approach usable in the future.

Traversing lesions. Localizing and marking the lesions to be crossed should be carried out immediately after puncture. This is best accomplished by comparing bony landmarks to the diagnostic arteriogram. Since laser recanalization may be performed in patients who have associated stenotic iliac arteries, the operator may be required to bypass such lesions in order to reach the occluded segment. The use of torque-controlled guidewires such as the Glidewire (Meditech, Inc., Watertown, MA) provides great precision for this task. In addition, multiplanar fluoroscopy, or digital fluoroscopy with road-mapping, can help provide more precise positioning. As in all angioplasty, a heparin bolus should be administered immediately after traversal of the lesions and before beginning laser recanalization. We usually administer this bolus intraarterially through the working catheter or sheath side arm, but intravenous administration is also acceptable.

Balloon choice. Various types of angioplasty balloons are available, and choice of balloon is somewhat controversial. High-pressure vs. low-pressure balloon, tip profile, shaft size and stiffness, and balloon shape have all been modified in some way or another. What is probably most important is to choose a device with which the operator is familiar and a balloon that is an appropriate size for the vessel being treated. Based on empirical observations and laboratory evaluation of angioplasty in the rabbit atherosclerosis model, most workers have chosen balloons that provided 30% overdilatation in an effort to reduce restenosis rate [5]. However, recent trials in coronary angioplasty (admittedly in very different vessels than arteries of the lower extremity) demonstrated an increased acute rethrombosis rate secondary to arterial dissection from overdilatation [6]. There are no hard clinical data that are useful in settling the issue. Our own approach is to choose a balloon of the size measured from the arteriogram (taking into account the presence of poststenotic dilatation). Since our radiographic system induces approximately 25% magnification during filming, this results in that much overdilatation.

Pressure measurements. Direct measurement of intraarterial peak systolic pressures above and below the lesion should be employed to determine the hemodynamic significance of the lesion to be treated and, more importantly, the results of treatment. These measurements are easily obtained in the aortoiliac vessels. Pretreatment gradients are not germane to the treatment of occlusive disease. Always leave a small-diameter guidewire across the area treated during repeat measurements after angioplasty, since the intimal disruptions produced by the balloon can prevent return to a proximal level and such attempts can result in displacement of the intimal flaps and occlusion of the vessel. The use of an 0.025 in. guidewire through a catheter tapered to 0.038 in. guides allows high-fidelity pressure measurement and is adequately stiff to guide the catheter safely.

For procedures in which pressures can be obtained accurately, the endpoint of the procedure should be obliteration of the gradient. The balloon catheter itself can be used for posttreatment pressure measurement. If a persistent gradient is demonstrated after treatment, the catheter can be withdrawn in small increments, with measurement of pressures at each increment. The point at which the pressure drops can be subjected to additional balloon inflations.

Postprocedure care. In general, heparin is not used in the postprocedure period for patients undergoing iliac angioplasty, since the incidence of immediate failure is extremely low in these patients. The average patient can be treated with overnight bed rest, and some workers, using small-diameter catheters, are even performing iliac angioplasty on short-stay outpatients. Where totally occluded segments of vessel are being recanalized, overnight heparin treatment may be appropriate.

Percutaneous Techniques for Infrainguinal Lesions

The treatment of infrainguinal disease has always been technically more demanding than is aortoiliac angioplasty, and its use for total occlusions has been less successful both initially and in the long term [7]. The new techniques have added to the technical complexity of treating this group of patients, while extending the population for whom angioplasty is suitable.

Access. Antegrade puncture of the common femoral artery is the single most difficult technique to learn as part of infrainguinal angioplasty. It is made more difficult because the position is awkward, selection of the puncture site more difficult, pathway of the artery less predictable, and the abdominal wall gets in the way in the obese patient. Once the common femoral artery is accessed, successfully cannulating the superficial femoral artery is often challenging because the natural tendency of guidewires introduced into the femoral artery is to travel posteriorly, toward the profunda femoris (see Fig. 3–1). This tendency can be overcome by several maneuvers: 1) Rotate the patient into the contralateral oblique and use an angled catheter or torque guide to search the anterior surface of the vessel or 2) place the leg into the frog lateral position, which changes the relative positions of the superficial femoral artery (SFA) and profunda to make SFA cannulation more likely [8].

Once the SFA is successfully catheterized, manipulation of catheters and guidewires may be hampered by the angulation of the introduction sheath produced by the patient's abdominal wall, especially in large patients (see Fig. 3–2). Both the laser probe and balloon catheter are susceptible to this problem. Fluoroscopy at the puncture site may be necessary to avoid puncturing the introduction sheath, and it may be necessary for the assistant to flatten the abdomen, reducing the angulation.

Because of the smaller size of the vessel, routine heparinization of the patient is begun as soon as successful entry has been accomplished. We employ a routine bolus of 5,000 IU given through the arterial catheter, but a dose based on patient weight is chosen by other workers.

Hemostasis at the end of the procedure can be more difficult. Because the skin incision is often high on the abdominal wall, there may not be bone against which to achieve adequate compression. It should be remembered that, unlike retrograde femoral puncture, in which the artery is punctured cephalad to the skin incision, the puncture is caudad in SFA angioplasty. Positioning of the fingers during compression must be adjusted appropriately. If puncture above the ligament is made because of a high origin of the SFA, bleeding into the pelvis can occur without formation of a hematoma, which goes unrecognized until the patient becomes hypotensive. The presence of a persistent tachycardia after the procedure, or an ongoing volume requirement, should suggest this complication.

Traversing lesions. Marking the site(s) of the lesions is equally important in infrainguinal procedures. It is more easily accomplished because blood is flowing toward, rather than away from, the areas to be treated. Our preference is to use radiopaque markers clipped to the drapes, but a radiopaque ruler can be placed adjacent to the extremity instead. In general, because of slower flow, and because the parts are thinner, and thus fluoroscopic visualization better, it is easier to traverse stenotic lesions of the SFA and popliteal arteries because their details can be better seen. The techniques and equipment employed are similar to those for the iliac vessels. It is often helpful to internally and/or externally rotate the extremity to improve orientation of the lesions. Some sort of torquing device, either catheter or guidewire, will be very useful. I prefer the Eisenberg torque guide (Elecath, Inc.), but the small (.014–.018 in.) so-called coronary wires are favored by many authors and the Glidewire is also useful here.

Techniques for passing the laser probe through lesions are described in chapters 4–10. Once the lesions have been passed, it may still be difficult, despite the creation of a laser-probe channel, to pass a balloon catheter through the lesions. Several techniques may help. The first is to dilate proximal lesions that may be preventing the catheter from advancing. The use of a Van Andel-type long-tapered PTFE dilating catheter (Cook, Inc.) will often allow smooth passage of the balloon. Lower profile balloons, with longer tapers, are also helpful. Using early laser probes, which were often then used as guidewires, it could be difficult to replace the probe with a stiffer guidewire. The newer catheter probes that are just becoming available can be manipulated over a guidewire, so that stiffer wires can be employed. Careful management of the puncture site, with flattening of any kinks in the introduction sheath, may also reduce friction and enhance passage of the balloon.

Special attention should be paid to the presence of spasm, which occurs in 10–20% of patients undergoing infrain-

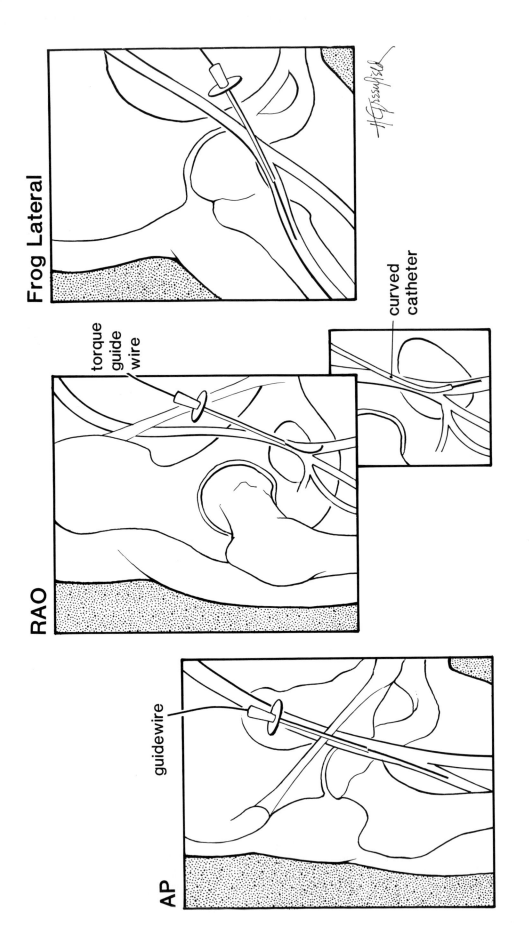

Fig. 3–1. Methods for cannulating the SFA during antegrade puncture. Left: Guidewires introduced during antegrade puncture tend to enter the profunda femoris because the needle points posteriorly. Middle: By lifting the ipsilateral hip, the profunda bifurcation is seen in profile. Depressing the needle hub may allow the guidewire to enter the SFA origin, but, if not, a torque wire or curved catheter can be used to select the anterior SFA. Right: The frog lateral position (leg abducted and externally rotated) can also be useful, since the puncture needle then tends to point toward the SFA rather than toward the profunda, increasing the chance that the guidewire will enter the SFA.

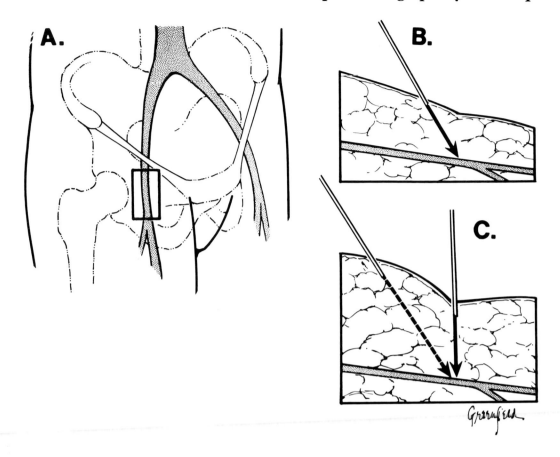

Fig. 3–2. Effect of body habitus on skin incision placement and catheter track. **A,** Desired area of entry into common femoral artery (rectangle). **B,** In the thin patient, when the skin incision is made about a few centimeters above the projected site of entry into the artery, the pathway of the catheter through soft tissue is short and the entry into the vessel is at an oblique angle. **C,** In the obese patient, in order to make an oblique entry into the vessel, the skin incision must be made relatively cephalad to the expected entry site. The pathway through the soft tissue may therefore be so long as to make puncture of the vessel difficult (dashed arrow). In addition, if care is not taken to adjust the position of compression after catheter removal, there is a likelihood of significant hematoma formation. If the skin incision is placed more caudad, the angle of entry into the vessel is almost vertical (solid arrow), causing kinking of the sheath and making the passage of catheters and guidewires much more difficult.

guinal angioplasty. We prefer intraarterial administration of nitroglycerin in 50 μm boluses, but others have used sublingual Nifedipine or ATP [9]. Local thromboemboli can be treated with acute thrombolytic infusions, as can acute reclosure of the angioplasty.

Balloon choice. Criteria for balloon choice are similar to those employed in other vessels. No special issues arise in femoropopliteal laser angioplasty.

Endpoint determination. Because of the smaller size of the vessels involved compared to the catheter size, and the necessity to measure pressures with the catheter across the lesion, pressure measurement, in general, is not useful in infrainguinal angioplasty. Arteriography of the treated area, using DSA, small-format serial films, or conventional serial films, is used, and multiple projections may be required. As in pressure measurement, leaving a small-diameter (0.025 in.)

guidewire through the treated area prevents disastrous results from attempting to recross lesions. The return of pulses previously absent can be used as a means of evaluating results, since the visual appearance of the vessel is often somewhat misleading.

Once the decision has been made that the lesions have been adequately treated, a full study of the extremity distal to the treatment site must be performed to demonstrate patency and exclude limb-threatening peripheral embolic occlusion.

Postprocedure care. Because, in general, the vessels are smaller in diameter, and often have more diseased segments treated, most workers have adopted a policy of heparinization for 24 h after the procedure, but no controlled studies have been performed that confirm the utility of this procedure. Since the patient has already had a bolus of heparin, we simply begin a continuous drip of heparin at 800–1,000 IU/h, checking the partial thromboplastin time (PTT) at 4 h and adjusting the dosage up or down to keep the PTT prolonged to 1.5–2 times baseline. The heparin is generally discontinued after 24 h of treatment.

Most workers advocate the use of antiplatelet agents such as ASA or Persantine or both. They may be omitted if the patient cannot tolerate the medication. The dose of ASA is generally 325 mg/day; recent studies suggest that smaller doses may be advantageous (M. Bettmann, unpublished data). Early recommendations that patients be treated with warfarin to prolong patency have never been shown to be valid.

Managing the Popliteal and Tibial Vessels

Treatment of atherosclerosis of the popliteal artery is similar to the treatment of the more proximal superficial artery in terms of techniques, balloon choices, and so forth. However, it must be handled with conservatism, since damage to the popliteal artery is much more difficult to manage surgically than is damage to the more proximal lower extremity arteries [10]. Also, surgical bypass to the tibial vessels is more difficult to perform and requires the presence of an adequate saphenous vein, since artificial conduits have very unfavorable patency rates [11], so that a mishap during angioplasty may be more likely to lead to amputation.

In the scope of this publication, tibial vessel disease will be managed largely with the laser probe, since it is able to provide an adequate lumen without the use of a balloon catheter. It should be noted, however, that balloon systems are available for this purpose that are similar to those used in coronary angioplasty and employ small diameter balloons placed coaxially. There is no large series of balloon procedures with long followup, so that the success rates and patency rates of this approach are not well documented.

CONCLUSIONS

From a technical standpoint, laser-assisted angioplasty is performed in a manner similar to conventional balloon angioplasty. Indeed, in many ways, the laser probes or laser catheters are simply more sophisticated guidewires than we have had before. Careful attention to the well-defined principles of balloon angioplasty will produce favorable results from the patients in whom laser angioplasty is attempted.

REFERENCES

1. Dotter CT, Judkins MP: Transluminal treatment of arteriosclerotic obstruction. Circulation 30:654–670, 1964.
2. Gruntzig AR: Die percutane transluminale Rekanalisation chronischer Arterienvershlusse mit einer neuen Dilatations technik. Baden-Baden: G. Witzstrick Verlag, 1977.
3. Chesebro JH, Lam Y, Badimon L, Fuster V: Restenosis after arterial angioplasty, a hemorrheologic response. Am J Cardiol 60:10b–16b, 1987.
4. Dietrich EB, Timbadia E, Bahadir I, Cohen K, Zenzen S: Argon laser assisted peripheral angioplasty. Vasc Surg 22:77–87, 1988.
5. LeVeen R, Flood B, Moore B, Wolfe G: Balloon oversizing reduces restenosis following angioplasty in atherosclerotic rabbit model. Invest Radiol (Supp. 18) 21:9, 1986 (abstract).
6. Douglas JS, King SB III, Roubin GS: Influence of the methodology of percutaneous transluminal coronary angioplasty on restenosis. Am J Cardiol 60:29b–31b, 1987.
7. Murray RR, Hewes RC, White RI, Mitchell SE, Auster M, Chang R, Kadir S, Kinnison ML, Kaufman SL: Long-segment femoro-popliteal stenoses: Is angioplasty a boon or a bust? Radiology 162:473–479, 1987.
8. Greenfield AJ: Percutaneous transluminal angioplasty of the femoral, popliteal, and tibial vessels. In Athanasoulis CA (ed): Interventional Radiology. Philadelphia: Saunders, 1982.
9. Krepel VM, van Andel GJ, van Erp WFM, Breslau PJ: Percutaneous transluminal angioplasty of the femoropopliteal artery: Initial and long-term results. Radiology 156:325–328, 1985.
10. Imperato A, Spencer FC: Peripheral arterial disease. In Schwartz SI (ed): Principles of Surgery. New York: McGraw-Hill, 1979.
11. Darling RC, Linton RR: Durability of femoropopliteal reconstructions. Am J Surg 123:472–479, 1972.

4. Laser Thermal Angioplasty: Equipment and Techniques

Timothy A. Sanborn, M.D.

INTRODUCTION

In this chapter, the short, 5-year development of the equipment and techniques used in laser thermal angioplasty will be reviewed and an attempt will be made to summarize the current "state of the art" of this rapidly evolving procedure. As will become readily apparent, there already have been significant changes and modifications in both the laser procedure and the actual laser devices. Techniques and equipment will continue to change in the near future. However, this chapter and those to follow should give the reader a good background in the equipment and techniques of the laser thermal angioplasty.

EQUIPMENT

Sheaths

With the development of flexible fiberoptics for transmission of laser energy, it became apparent in the early 1980s that it may be possible to harness laser energy for percutaneous, nonsurgical removal of atheroma or thrombus in recanalization of obstructive arteries. In initial clinical trials, bare fiberoptics were advanced through the central lumen of angiographic or balloon catheters in order to gain close approximation to peripheral arterial lesions [1,2]. In experimental studies [3–5] with the laser-probe device, however, it was found that larger, 2.0 mm diameter tips could create wider channels. Unfortunately, advancement of these 2.0-mm diameter tips through a guiding catheter was not possible. Therefore, a conventional 7–8 F sheath with a side arm for injection of contrast was used to allow passage of the early laser-probe devices into the superficial femoral artery via an antegrade puncture (see chap. 3).

Choice of sheaths. Over the past 3 years, we have used a number of sheaths during laser thermal angioplasty procedures. These include those manufactured by Cook, Cordis, and USCI.

Sheath qualities. The two main qualities we have found important in a sheath for antegrade punctures are 1) hemostasis and 2) stiffness. The hemostatic issue is different in laser thermal angioplasty as compared to conventional angioplasty in that the sheath has to have a large internal luminal diameter to accommodate a 2.0 mm and now a 2.5 mm diameter metal probe and also be capable of maintaining a good hemostatic seal around a small 300 μm fiberoptic. In our experience, the present Cordis sheath with its bivalve design has the best hemostasis, with the Cook sheath being second best. Current USCI sheaths cannot maintain good hemostasis around this small fiberoptic and other sheaths with Tuohy-Borst adapters are too cumbersome.

The antegrade puncture, as opposed to the retrograde approach, often requires advancement through considerable subcutaneous tissue—particularly in obese patients (chap. 3). This approach requires a stiffer sheath and introducer than that commonly used in the retrograde approach. In our hands, the Cordis sheath has unfortunately been too thin and the dilator too small for the sheath, such that the sheath has torn on several occasions in antegrade approaches. This can cause a tramatic arteriotomy, and a local surgical repair has been required on a few occasions. For this reason, we currently consider the Cook sheath as the best overall sheath for antegrade punctures. Obviously, the Cordis sheath can be strengthened and the homeostatic valve on the Cook sheath improved from their present designs.

Early Laser Probes

The initial laser-probe devices used clinically in peripheral arteries consisted of 2.0 mm diameter elliptical metal caps placed on a 300 μm core-diameter fiberoptic. In order to gain clinical experience with this device, very simple straightforward stenoses were attempted first. For safety reasons in the first few cases, the device was passed over a small coronary guidewire in order to

Laser Angioplasty, pages 21–28
© 1989 Alan R. Liss, Inc.

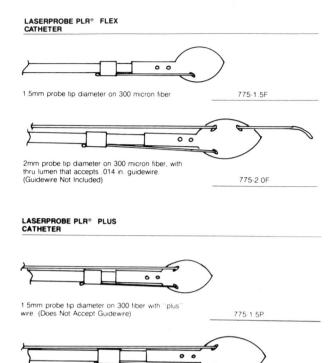

LASERPROBE PLR® FLEX
CATHETER

1.5mm probe tip diameter on 300 micron fiber   775-1.5F

2mm probe tip diameter on 300 micron fiber, with
thru lumen that accepts .014 in. guidewire.
(Guidewire Not Included)   775-2.0F

LASERPROBE PLR® PLUS
CATHETER

1.5mm probe tip diameter on 300 fiber with "plus"
wire. (Does Not Accept Guidewire)   775-1.5P

2.0mm probe tip diameter on 300 micron fiber with
"plus" wire.   775-2.0P

Fig. 4–1. First-generation laser-probe devices. Top: 1.5 mm and 2.0 mm diameter "flex" laser probes. Bottom: Similar "plus" laser-probe devices. (Figure courtesy of Trimedyne, Inc., Santa Ana, CA).

help prevent vessel perforation. An eccentric guidewire channel allowed for this "over-the-wire" technique.

Probe detachment. In the second clinical case, a popliteal artery total occlusion, probe detachment from the fiberoptic occurred. Subsequent to this experience, a short safety wire was added to all devices to prevent loss of the metal tip should tip detachment occur. Perhaps more important was the incorporation of a larger 0.014 in. "plus" anchor wire that added stability to the union between the fiberoptic and the metal tip. The wire ran along the entire intravascular length of the fiberoptic so that should the finer safety wire fail the probe could still be retrieved.

First-generation laser probes. Diagrams of these "first-generation" laser-probe designs are shown in Figure 4–1. Some investigators preferred the flexibility of the "flex" probe, whereas others preferred the added axial stiffness of the "plus" probes. On occasion, smaller, 1.5 mm laser probes with a lower profile were found to be able to recanalize occlusions when a larger 2.0 mm device was unsuccessful (Fig. 4–2). As observed experimentally [3–5], larger probes created larger channels. Thus, if a lesion could be crossed with a 1.5 mm

device, then the 2.0 mm device was usually tried in order to obtain the larger luminal diameter and the maximal amount of laser recanalization. This concept later led to the development of even larger 2.5 mm laser-probe devices that could still be introduced percutaneously to an 8 F sheath.

LASER-PROBE TECHNIQUE

Technique Development

Historically, the technique of laser thermal angioplasty was developed and first shown to be effective in an atherosclerotic rabbit iliac artery model [3,5] prior to clinical use. Dr. Hany Hussein (Trimedyne, Inc., Santa Ana, CA) developed an argon laser fiberoptic with a simple metal cap on its tip [6] to protect the fiberoptic from "burning up" if brought in contact with tissue during laser-pulse delivery. Ironically, the metal tip was later found to have several functions (radiopacity, a rounded blunt tapered tip, and circumferential distribution of thermal energy) that contributed significantly to the success of the device in recanalizing total occlusions.

Stationary laser-pulse delivery. Interestingly, in the early animal studies of this device, the laser procedure consisted of laser pulses of 6 W of argon laser energy delivered for 2 s duration to a 0.9 mm laser probe while the device was maintained in a "stationary" position in the iliac artery [3]. With this technique, angiographic improvement in luminal diameter could be demonstrated. For tubular lesions, two pulses approximately 1 cm apart were used to create two areas of increased luminal diameter (Fig. 4–3).

The first clinical case with a 2.0 mm laser-probe device was performed successfully with this "stationary" laser-probe technique (Fig. 4–4). As mentioned above, for safety reasons, a small coronary guidewire was first passed through the lesion to maintain access to the distal vessel should spasm or thrombosis occur (Fig. 4–4, top right). Then, the 2.0 mm laser probe was brought up in contact with the high-grade eccentric stenosis, and gentle mechanical recanalization or "Dottering" of this lesion was not found possible. However, while maintaining gentle pressure on the lesion and using 6 W of laser energy delivered for a total of 16 s, significant improvement in the lumen could be achieved and no further resistance to passage through the lesion was felt (Fig. 4–4, bottom left). The lesion was then further dilated with subsequent conventional balloon angioplasty (Fig. 4–4, bottom right).

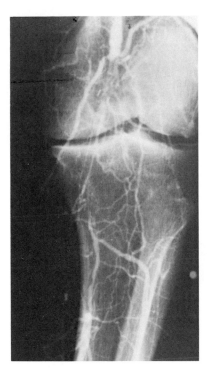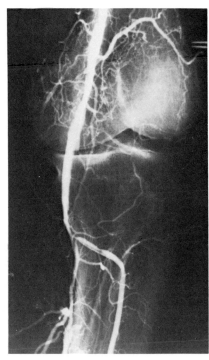

Fig. 4–2. Angiogram of an 8 cm popliteal artery occlusion that could not be crossed with a 2.0 mm laser probe but could be recanalized with a 1.5 mm laser probe and subsequently dilated with conventional balloon angioplasty.

In the second clinical case, the stationary laser delivery technique proved to be disastrous when the metal tip became adherent to the arterial wall and detached from the fiberoptic while attempting to recanalize the last 1 cm of a 4 cm hard fibrocellular popliteal artery occlusion. Whether tip detachment was related to excessive pressure and "buckling" at the weak union between the fiberoptic and the metal tip or to a pulling apart of the fiberoptic from the metal cap during an attempt to withdraw the device after adherence was noted could not be determined, but it was clear that adherence had to be avoided and a stronger improved delivery system was needed.

The "constant-motion" technique. Without a stronger fiberoptic metal tip system readily available, a "constant-motion" technique of moving the metal tip back and forth in the lesion during laser-pulse delivery and cooling down was used in the third clinical case to avoid the problem of adherence to the vessel wall. Using this technique, successful laser recanalization of a subtotal superficial femoral artery stenosis was achieved and followed by subsequent balloon angioplasty (Fig. 4–5). With the incorporation of this constant-motion technique into all subsequent laser thermal angioplasty procedures and the improvements in the laser delivery system (safety wire and 0.014 in. "plus" wire), the risk

of probe detachment was virtually eliminated.

The rapidity with which the laser probe is moved back and forth through the lesion may determine how much of the lesion is vaporized versus how much is mechanically dilated. The more rapid the probe is advanced through the lesion, the more likely "mechanical" recanalization is likely to result. Therefore, one has to temper the desire to move rapidly and avoid adherence with the goal of vaporizing and/or compressing [7] as much tissue as possible. I have found a slow but gradual back-and-forth motion over a few centimeters of length of vessel with 3–5 s laser pulses to be most effective. After each 3–5 s pulse, I intermittently inject contrast solution through the side arm of the sheath to monitor progress of the laser probe until the occlusion has been completely recanalized.

Tip angulation by wire shaping. Occasionally, in tortuous lesions, or at bifurcations in the artery, some angulation of this straight but flexible fiberoptic and the rigid metal tip is necessary. As described above, early in this clinical trial, a 0.014 in. guidewire was placed along the side of the fiberoptic to add stability to the union between the metal tip and the fiberoptic. By shaping a gentle curve in the distal portion of this wire, a curve can also be maintained in the fiberoptic such that the metal tip can be rotated 360° in a fashion similar to

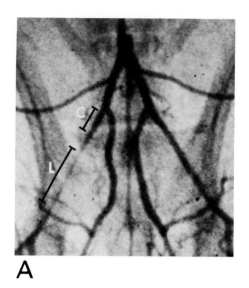
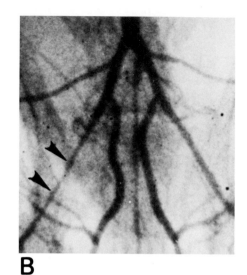

Fig. 4–3. Angiographic example with laser probe demonstrating **A,** a long tubular 90% mid-right iliac artery lesion (L) relative to a proximal control segment (C). **B,** Lesion was treated with 2 pulses (6 W, 2 s)

1 cm apart that resulted in 30% residual stenosis (arrows). Reproduced with permission of T.A. Sanborn et al. and the American College of Cardiology (Journal of the American College of Cardiology 5:934, 1985).

torque guidewires. Care must be taken, however, to be sure that this angulation is not too acute as the curve is fixed and may make further recanalization of a straight portion of the artery more difficult. Biplane fluoroscopy or use of multiple fluoroscopic views aids in the use of

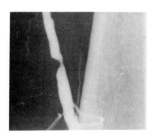
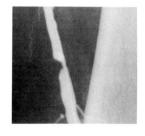
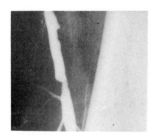
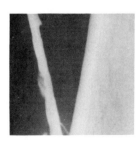

Fig. 4–4. Top left panel: 70–80% high-grade eccentric superficial femoral artery stenosis. Top right panel: 2.0 mm laser probe advanced over a coronary guidewire up to the stenosis. Bottom left panel: Stenosis reduced to an approximately 50% residual stenosis after laser thermal angioplasty. Bottom right panel: Final angiographic result after subsequent balloon angioplasty.

these angled probes. The ability to release the angulation, as in a tip-deflecting wire, would be a useful alternative to improve the steerability of the device in the future.

Balloon advancement over the probe. In extremely difficult or tortuous lesions, another technique that has proven useful is the advancement of the balloon angioplasty catheter over the fiberoptic and the 0.014 in. wire once the lesion has been crossed. In this situation, instead of recrossing the lesion with a guidewire that can cause a dissection, the fiberoptic and the wire actually serves as the guidewire for the balloon catheter. This technique has been quite helpful, particularly in diffusely diseased vessels. The sterile portion of the disposable fiberoptic does have to be cut about 2 m from the distal end in order to disconnect it from the nonsterile proximal end that is attached to the laser generator. A laser-probe catheter with a central lumen large enough to accept a 0.038 in. guidewire is now under investigation (Sanborn et al., unpublished results) and should further improve this exchange.

Glazing. Knowing that balloon angioplasty often leaves the vessel surface fractured and split after dilatation and that this could be a nidus for platelet accumulation, thrombosis, smooth muscle cell proliferation, and abrupt closure and/or restenosis, a concept proposed by Myler et al. [8] was that of using the laser probe after balloon angioplasty to "glaze" or smooth the roughened inner surface of the vessel wall after balloon dilatation. Although there have been a

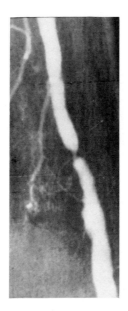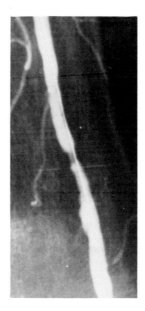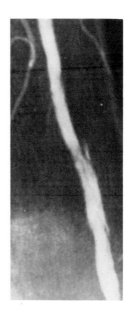

Fig. 4–5. Left panel: 80–90% superficial femoral artery stenosis. Middle panel: Improved angiographic result after a 2.0 mm laser probe is advanced through the stenosis using the "constant-motion" technique over a coronary guidewire. Right panel: End result after subsequent balloon angioplasty.

few clinical examples suggestive of some angiographic improvement (see chap. 6), the pathophysiological mechanism of glazing is unknown. Conceptually, there is a question as to what effect a 2.0 mm or even a 2.5 mm laser-probe device that functions as a "contact" device will have in a vessel dilated with a 5 mm or 6 mm balloon catheter. Theoretically, the probe should slide through the dilated segment without making much contact with the vessel wall. Although there has been some experimental evidence that a laser-balloon catheter may be able to "seal" intimal flaps and decrease "elastic recoil" after balloon dilatation [9], to date, experimental studies with existing laser-probe devices have failed to demonstrate significant angiographic or histologic evidence of successful laser sealing [10]. In addition, the risk of mechanical or thermal perforation by the laser probe may actually be greater after balloon-induced fracture of the vessel wall. The use of larger fixed or expandable laser devices used "over the wire" could improve the ability to seal such dissections, but further studies are warranted to examine this intriguing concept.

MEDICATION

As in conventional balloon angioplasty, we still do not have a standard antiplatelet or anticoagulant regimen for laser thermal angioplasty. As evident from some of the other contributors to this volume, several different regimens may be used. Unlike coronary angioplasty where a femoral sheath can be left in place overnight while systematic heparin is administered, leaving a sheath in place above a recanalized and dilated femoropopliteal lesion can significantly reduce blood flow, cause stagnation, and probably contribute to a higher early reclosure rate.

Initially, our drug regimen consisted of 325 mg of aspirin prior to the procedure and 5,000 U of heparin administered interarterially after the sheath had been placed. After the angioplasty, the sheaths were pulled immediately to remove obstruction to blood flow, and if a significant hematoma was not present, systemic heparin was administered overnight. After several complications of expanding groin hematomas, we discontinued administering systemic heparin overnight. The trade-off with this approach is that the risk of early thrombotic reclosure may be higher. Obviously, more research is needed to investigate the incidence of significant groin hematomas and early thrombotic closures with different regimens. Perhaps a simple local femoral cutdown and arteriotomy repair postangioplasty would decrease the risk of significant groin hematoma and allow for the potential benefit of safer systemic heparinization overnight.

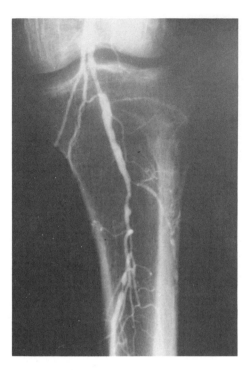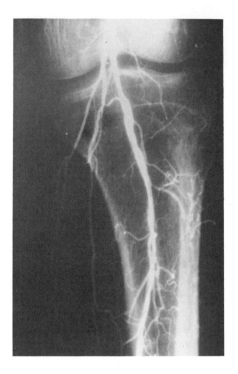

Fig. 4–6.   Example of sole laser thermal angioplasty of a 12 cm popliteal artery stenosis and a 1 cm anterior tibial artery stenosis performed with a 2.5 mm central lumen laser-probe catheter advanced over a 0.035 in. guidewire. The anterior tibial artery stenosis could only be crossed with a coronary guidewire, and the laser probe advanced over this smaller guidewire.

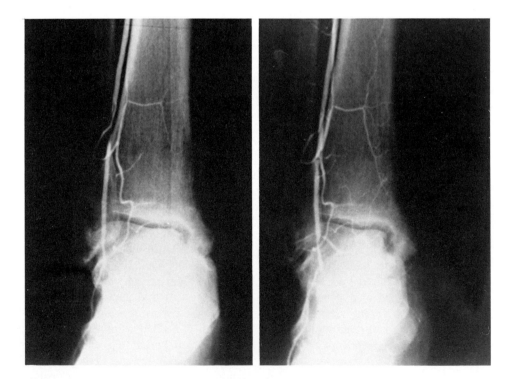

Fig. 4–7.   Example of sole laser thermal angioplasty of a 3 cm distal anterior tibial artery stenosis near the ankle with a 2.5 mm central lumen laser-probe catheter advanced over a 0.035 in. guidewire.

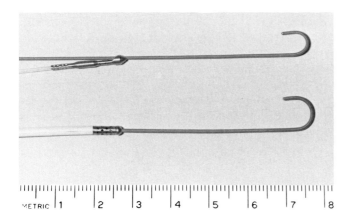

Fig. 4–8. Example of 2.5 mm "over-the-wire" laser probes. Top: Eccentric probe over a 0.035 in. guidewire. Bottom: Central lumen laser-probe catheter over a 0.038 in. guidewire.

"SECOND-GENERATION" LASER PROBES

Larger Diameter

Early clinical experience with 1.5 mm and 2.0 mm laser probes confirmed the experimental observation [3–5] that larger laser probes produced larger recanalized channels on angiography. This observation is most likely due to the fact that the mechanism of action of this device is by "contact" with tissue and that thermal compression as well as vaporization [7] is involved in the pathophysiology in this technique.

Therefore, the manufacturer was asked to make laser probes larger than 2.0 mm. Apparently, a 2.5 mm device is just about the maximum size that can currently be inserted through a sheath and heated with a 14 W argon laser generator. Larger, 3.5 mm and 5.0 mm devices have been introduced with a surgical cutdown and heated with a more powerful Nd:YAG laser.

Sole Laser Thermal Angioplasty

In our experience, the 2.5 mm device is capable of opening larger channels than was possible with the first-generation devices. Furthermore, in 18 cases, we have been able to perform sole laser thermal angioplasty of distal popliteal and tibial arteries without the need for subsequent balloon angioplasty (Figs. 4–6, 4–7). Sole laser thermal angioplasty may allow for a smoother luminal surface that is less likely to develop abrupt closure and restenosis than is laser-assisted balloon angioplasty or balloon angioplasty alone as seen in experimental studies [5].

"Over-the-Wire" Laser Probes

While some of the early laser-probe cases were performed over a small coronary guidewire, in general, these guidewires were too small and did not provide adequate axial strength or "stiffness" for use

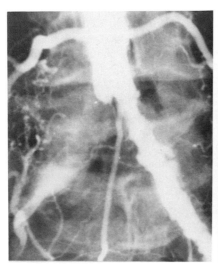
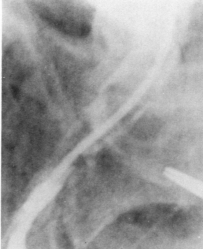
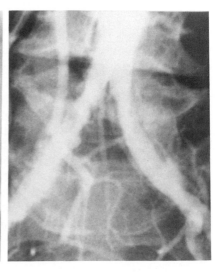

Fig. 4–9. Angiograms of a 3 cm right iliac artery occlusion (left panel) that required an axillary approach because of an inadequate femoral artery pulse. The 2.5 mm eccentric probe was tried first over a guidewire, but could not even be advanced to the distal aorta because of subclavian artery and aortic tortuosity. A 2.5 mm central lumen laser-probe catheter could be advanced very easily over a standard guidewire to recanalize this iliac artery occlusion (middle panel) for subsequent angioplasty (right panel).

in larger peripheral arteries. What was needed was a device that could be advanced over a stiffer 0.035–0.038 in. guidewire (Fig. 4–8). In addition, from experience in coronary arteries and a few cases in peripheral arteries (Fig. 4–9), we learned that an eccentric probe or "monorail"-type device with a small channel only through the side of the metal tip did not slide very well back and forth over the guidewire. This was due to excessive friction through the narrow channel and poor coaxiality between the independent fiberoptic and guidewire. Rather, the fiberoptic and the guidewire would often have to be moved together as a unit. This technique has, on occasion, caused guidewire-induced distal arterial spasm in peripheral arteries. As demonstrated in Figure 4–9, I have also had difficulty advancing the eccentric probe over a 0.035–0.038 in. guidewire in tortuous vessels.

The 2.5 mm laser probe with a central lumen (Fig. 4–8, bottom) solves these problems of trackability and is actually a catheter with a central channel for a guidewire. The central lumen can also be used for distal contrast injection (see Fig. 4–9), and this capability has been extremely useful for visualization of distal tibial and peroneal artery lesions that are difficult to opacify with injections through the sheath in the common femoral artery.

FUTURE PERIPHERAL DEVICES AND TECHNIQUE

This chapter represents a very brief overview of current laser thermal angioplasty devices: some of these such as the laser-probe catheter have been only recently approved by the FDA (June 1988). These devices will most certainly undergo significant changes in the future. To date, the majority of peripheral laser-probe cases have been performed with argon-heated laser probes; however, this may be changing over to Nd:YAG-heated laser probes as the more powerful Nd:YAG laser will be capable of heating larger laser probes. Expandable and rotational laser probes are also now being tested in the animal laboratory in an attempt to provide sole laser thermal angioplasty without the need for subsequent balloon angioplasty in large peripheral arteries.

In terms of laser thermal angioplasty technique, it is interesting to note that the actual laser procedure itself has remained relatively unchanged. Although there may be some individual operator variations, the "constant-

motion" technique has been used uniformly by all investigators with little change in over 3 years. It has also been interesting to note as other laser devices have begun early clinical trials that fluoroscopic recordings of laser procedures with these devices also employed this same constant-motion technique. Whether the constant-motion technique will remain the same with newer devices or prove feasible in tortuous coronary arteries remains to be determined.

REFERENCES

1. Ginsberg R, Wexler L, Mitchell RS, Profitt D: Percutaneous transluminal laser angioplasty for treatment of peripheral vascular disease: Clinical experience with 16 patients. Radiology 156:619–624, 1985.

2. Cumberland DC, Tayler DI, Procter AE: Laser-assisted percutaneous angioplasty: Initial clinical experience in peripheral arteries. Clin Radiol 37:423–428, 1986.

3. Sanborn TA, Faxon DP, Haudenschild C, Ryan TJ: Experimental angioplasty: Circumferential distribution of laser thermal energy with a laser probe. J Am Coll Cardiol 5:934–938, 1985.

4. Abela GS, Fenech A, Crea F, Conti F, Conti CR: "Hot tip": Another method of laser vascular recanalization. Lasers Surg Med 5:327–335, 1985.

5. Sanborn TA, Haudenschild CC, Faxon DP, Garber GR, Ryan TJ: Angiographic and histologic consequences of laser thermal angioplasty: Comparison with balloon angioplasty. Circulation 75:1281–1284, 1987.

6. Hussein H: A novel fiberoptic laser probe for treatment of occlusive vessel disease. Optical Laser Technol Med 605:59–66, 1986.

7. Welch AJ, Bradley AB, Torres JH, Motamedi M, Ghidori JJ, Pearse JA, Hussein H, O'Rourke RA: Laser probe ablation of normal and atheroclerotic human aortic in vitro: A first thermographic and histologic analysis. Circulation 76:1353–1363, 1987.

8. Myler RK, Cumberland DC, Clark DA, Stertzer SH, Tatpati DA, Sen Sarma PK: High and low power thermal laser angioplasty for total occlusions and restenosis in man (abstract). Circulation 76:IV–230, 1987.

9. Spears JR: Percutaneous transluminal coronary angioplasty restenosis: Potential prevention with laser balloon angioplasty. Am J Cardiol 60:61B–64B, 1987.

10. Stroh JA, Sanborn TA, Haudenschild CC: Experimental argon laser thermal angioplasty as an adjunct to balloon angioplasty (abstract). J Am Coll Cardiol 11:108A, 1988.

5. Initial Multicenter Training and Experience With 1.5- and 2.0-mm Peripheral Laser Probes

Timothy A. Sanborn, M.D.

INTRODUCTION

The initial clinical experience with laser thermal angioplasty in peripheral arteries [1–3] suggests that this technique is a safe and effective adjunct to balloon angioplasty in that it can recanalize lesions that previously could not be treated by conventional means [1]. However, these initial results were obtained at two centers with extensive experimental [4,5] and prior clinical experience with argon laser angioplasty [6]. One question that needed to be answered was whether this new technique could be easily learned and used safely and effectively by physicians experienced in conventional peripheral balloon angioplasty techniques. The present chapter will address this issue, discuss physician training in this new technique, and summarize the initial multicenter experience from ten institutions [7].

PHYSICIAN TRAINING

Physician training was key in the development of this initial experience in as safe a manner as possible. After the technique had been developed in over 40 patients at two centers (see chap. 6), eight additional investigators with extensive experience in peripheral balloon angioplasty were trained through a combination of the following: 1) obtaining knowledge of laser safety, laser physics, and laser-tissue interaction; 2) gaining "hands-on" experience in atherosclerotic rabbits or post-mortem specimens; 3) observing videotapes and/or actual "live" cases; and, finally, 4) clinical participation in several laser cases with one of the established investigators.

Today, more than 3 years after this initial experience, cardiovascular laser training remains a significant concern. Unfortunately, in some institutions, significant debate and in a few cases "turf battles" have developed over which physicians are best qualified to perform these procedures. In some instances, for political reasons, laser credentials have actually been denied to the best-qualified individuals. The cardiovascular area should not be any different from other areas of medicine and surgery in which lasers are used, and standards of practice have been developed according to the guidelines as established by the American Society of Laser Medicine and Surgery.

More important than attending a laser course or watching a few cases, however, is the need to be skilled in conventional peripheral balloon angioplasty and interventional radiology techniques. It has often been said that laser recanalization of a lesion is sometimes the easiest part of the angioplasty procedure. The antegrade puncture as well as the choice and handling of various guidewires and balloon catheters requires considerable experience that is unique to a vascular radiologist. Despite my own training in cardiac catheterization and coronary angioplasty, I have always performed our laser-assisted balloon angioplasty procedures in collaboration with one of my colleagues in radiology. This cooperation is the key in obtaining the best result with the lowest risk of complications for the patient. Most other successful cardiovascular laser centers have also developed similar types of collaborative approach to laser angioplasty, whether it be a cardiologist and a vascular radiologist working together with surgical consultation or a vascular surgeon teamed up with an interventional radiologist. The free exchange of different techniques and methods adds significantly to the overall likelihood of success.

THE MULTICENTER TRIAL

Between April 1985 and November 1986, laser-assisted balloon angioplasty was performed in 219 peripheral arteries in 208 patients at ten medical centers. These centers and their principal investigators are as follows:

Boston University Medical Center, Boston, MA.
    Timothy A. Sanborn, M.D., Alan J. Greenfield, M.D., Jon K. Guben, M.D.
Johns Hopkins Medical Center, Baltimore, MD.
    Robert I. White, M.D., Robert R. Murray, M.D.
Northern General Hospital, Sheffield, England.
    David C. Cumberland, M.D., Christopher L. Welch, M.D.

TABLE 5–1. Initial Angiographic and Clinical Results

Angioplasty category	No.	Mean lesion length (cm)	Angiographic success		Clinical success	
Possible	149	6.8	128	(86)	116	(78)
Stenosis	41		40	(98)	39	(95)
Occlusions	108		88	(81)	77	(71)
Impossible	70	11.7	44	(63)	39	(56)
Stenosis	4		4	(100)	4	(100)
Occlusions	66		40	(61)	35	(53)
Total	219	8.3	172	(79)	155	(71)

Nos. in parentheses represent percent success in each group.

St. Anne's Hospital, Chicago, IL.
    Amir Motarjeme, M.D.
St. Joseph's Hospital, Wichita, KS.
    Daniel Tapati, M.D.
St. Vincent's Hospital, Indianapolis, IN.
    Donald E. Schwarten, M.D.
Seton Medical Center, Daly City, CA.
    Richard K. Myler, M.D.
Stanford Medical Center, Palo Alto, CA.
    Robert Ginsberg, M.D.
Texas Heart Institute, Houston, TX.
    D. Richard Leachmann, M.D.
University of Arkansas Health Sciences Center, Little
    Rock, AK. *Ernest J. Ferris, M.D.,*
    Timothy C. McCowan, M.D.

The indications for angioplasty were severe claudication that was unresponsive to exercise therapy and pentoxifylline in 96 (44%) lesions and rest pain, nonhealing ulcer, or gangrene in 123 (56%) lesions. Nine straight iliac arteries and 210 femoropopliteal arteries were treated. There were 166 (76%) occlusions and 53 (24%) stenosis. Initial evaluation included a history and physical examination as well as a Doppler ankle-arm index (AAI), which was also used for follow-up after angioplasty. Patients were pretreated with oral aspirin (75 or 325 mg once a day) prior to the procedure. The majority of the procedures were performed via percutaneous arterial puncture of the ipsilateral femoral artery under local anesthesia [1–3].

In eight patients, either marked obesity or high-grade proximal superficial femoral artery disease precluded a safe percutaneous approach. In these cases, under local anesthesia and mild sedation, a small cutdown was made to expose the common femoral artery for direct arterial puncture and subsequent laser and balloon angioplasty through an 8.5 F sheath [2]. The results to be discussed were obtained with the first generation of 1.5 mm and 2.0 mm laser probes.

Lesion Classification

From previous assessment of the angiogram and/or by gentle probing at the proximal end of the occlusion with a guidewire (without an attempt to cross the lesion), all lesions were classified by the clinical investigator as to the probability of success by conventional peripheral balloon angioplasty (i.e., possible or impossible), as previously reported [5]. Prior failed attempts with conventional balloon angioplasty were considered in the impossible category. Altogether, 149 (68%) of these lesions were considered possible to treat by conventional balloon angioplasty, while almost one-third (70) of these lesions were impossible to treat by conventional balloon angioplasty (Table 5–1). The incidence of rest pain, ulcer, or gangrene in the possible and impossible categories was 52 and 66%, respectively.

Interpretation of Results

The results of laser-assisted balloon angioplasty were classified as follows:

Angiographic and clinical success. This was defined as an angiographic improvement in the luminal diameter to less than 50% residual stenosis, improvement of symptoms to the point where the patients could resume their desired life styles or limb salvage was achieved, improved pulse, and an increase in the Doppler AAI by greater than 0.15, as previously described [8–10].

Angiographic success but immediate clinical failure. In this group, improvement in the angiographic appearance was less than ideal (small luminal diameter, significant luminal irregularities). Symptoms were not relieved and the Doppler AAI did not increase.

Angiographic failure. Inability to cross the lesion with the laser-probe device or to improve the ap-

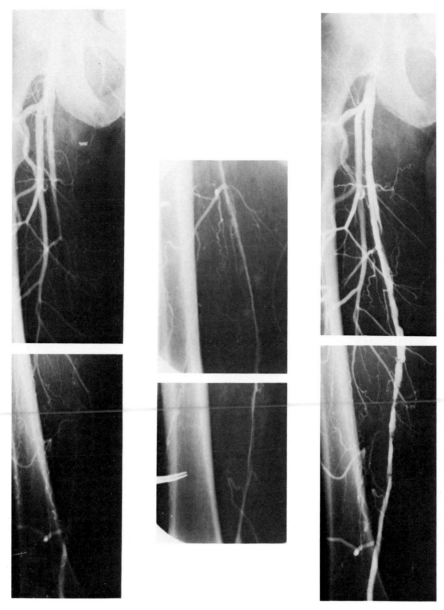

Fig. 5–1. Angiograms of a 15 cm right superficial femoral artery occlusion: (left panel) before treatment; (middle panel) after recanalization with six pulses (5-s duration) of 12 W of argon laser energy delivered to a 2.5 mm laser probe; (right panel) after dilatation with a 6 mm balloon catheter. Reproduced with permission of T.A. Sanborn et al. and the American Medical Association (Archives of Surgery, in press, 1989).

pearance of the lesion to less than 50% residual stenosis was considered an angiographic (technical) failure.

Acute Angiographic and Clinical Results

The overall initial angiographic clinical success for all 219 lesions was 71% with the likelihood of angioplasty success (possible or impossible) influencing im-

mediate technical and clinical success (Table 5–1). For lesions considered possible to treat by conventional balloon angioplasty, the clinical success rate of 78% is equal to or better than that reported in the literature for conventional balloon angioplasty [8–9]. In this series, clinical success was achieved in 39 of 41 (95%) stenoses and 77 of 108 (71%) total occlusions in this possible category.

Potentially, one of the most important benefits of laser thermal angioplasty is the ability to quickly and

TABLE 5–2. Incidence of Complications in 219 Arteries

Complications	Probe related %	Probe related No.	Procedure related %	Procedure related No.	Incidence with conventional balloon angioplasty Ref. 12 (%)	Incidence with conventional balloon angioplasty Ref. 13 (%)
Death	0	(0)	0	(0)	0.3	0
Emergency surgery	0	(0)	0	(0)	3.0	—
Embolization	0	(0)	2.7	(6)	1.5	5
Probe detachment	1.8	(4)	—	—	—	—
Groin hematoma	0	(0)	3.2	(7)	4	2
Infection	0	(0)	0	(0)	—	—
Perforation	4.1	(9)	4.6	(10)	—	0–3
Rupture	0	(0)	0	(0)	0.4	0–1
Spasm	0	(0)	1.8	(4)	—	0–5
Subintimal dissection	5.0	(11)	5.0	(11)	4	1

No. in parentheses represent no. complications in 219 patients.

safely recanalize lesions that are impossible to treat by conventional means. In particular, over one-half (56%) of those lesions that were not amenable to balloon angioplasty alone were successfully treated with laser-assisted balloon angioplasty.

Representative angiographic results of laser-assisted balloon angioplasty of a 15 cm right superficial femoral artery occlusion are shown in Figure 5–1. In this patient, the AAI rose from 0.46 to 1.06 after angioplasty.

Laser Parameters

In this study, the most commonly used laser-probe size was the 2.0 mm diameter metal tip. The average laser wattage was 10 W (range 4–13 W). Of particular note, the average laser delivery time to recanalize these lesions was only 24 s (range 5–113 s).

Complications

In this initial series, which represents an expansion from two initial clinical centers to a total of ten, the complications that arose from laser-assisted balloon angioplasty were minimal (Table 5–2). Most notable was that the perforation rate with this laser device was only 4.1% and there was no requirement for emergency bypass surgery. This perforation rate was only 2.1% in those lesions considered possible to treat by balloon angioplasty alone.

In a trial that represents not only the clinical development stage of a new device but also early operator "learning" experience, it is important to note that the incidence of various complications is no greater than that noted in two recent reports [11–12] of conventional balloon angioplasty (Table 5–2). One early concern with laser angioplasty was the incidence of perforation, which complicated early clinical trials [6,13]. In the present series, the 4.1% incidence of vessel perforation with no significant clinical sequelae is much lower than in previous clinical series using bare argon laser fiberoptics for peripheral laser angioplasty in which vessel perforation was noted in 2 of 15 (13%) [6] and 3 of 16 (19%) [13] vessels.

The decreased incidence of vessel perforation with this device is probably multifactorial. From a design standpoint, the rounded but tapered tip provides a blunt object that is less likely to mechanically perforate the artery compared with sharp, pointed fiberoptics [4]. Second, the metal probe has been shown to disperse thermal energy uniformly around the tip so as not to focus all laser energy in one spot [14]. Histologic analysis after the use of this device indicates a thermal effect around the entire luminal circumference of a diseased vessel [4]. Thus, dispersion and circumferential distribution of thermal energy rather than attempting to aim a narrow laser beam could also contribute to reduce perforation. Finally, vaporization of fibrofatty plaque with this laser probe device was possible at a lower temperature than for normal (elastic and collagen) tissue [14]; this may also contribute to reduce perforation.

Probe Detachment

Early in this clinical trial, probe-tip detachment from the fiberoptic occurred in four patients; all but one of these probes could be retrieved and removed. Subse-

TABLE 5-3. Learning Curve of Success and Complications

Clinical center	No.	Clinical success	Intimal dissection	Perforation
Boston University	19	16 (84)	0	0
Northern General Hospital	105	73 (70)	4 (3.8)	3 (2.9)
Other eight centers	95*	66 (69)	7 (7.4)	7 (7.4)

Nos. in parentheses represent percent of total attempts.
* Average of 12 per site.

quent to this early experience, a 0.014 in. safety (anchor) wire was incorporated into the device to add stability to the union between the fiberoptic and the metal tip and to prevent further probe detachment. This wire runs along the entire intravascular length of the fiberoptic so that should tip detachment occur the probe could be retrieved. In addition, by keeping the probe moving constantly during laser delivery and the cooling period, it was found that adherence to the vessel wall, one of the potential causes of probe detachment, was significantly reduced.

Learning Curve of Success and Complications

In this multicentered clinical trial, clinical success and incidence of complications improved considerably as the operator gained experience with the laser-probe device (Table 5-3). In terms of complications, the lowest incidence of perforations (0%) occurred at Boston University where extensive experiments and a "tactile" sense for the device had been gained from prior experimental studies in atherosclerotic rabbits and post-mortem specimens. However, clinical centers could also learn this technique and gain experience with the device quite rapidly without a high incidence of complication. For example, at Northern General Hospital, the incidence of perforation decreased from 1 in 14 patients (7%) to 2 in the first 40 patients (5%) and then 1 in the last 65 patients (1.5%).

CONCLUSIONS

In this multicenter series of 219 peripheral artery laser-assisted balloon angioplasty procedures, there is evidence that the process of laser thermal angioplasty with an argon laser-heated metal-capped fiberoptic allows for nonsurgical treatment of lesions difficult or impossible to treat by conventional means. The technique can be easily learned and performed without added risk compared to conventional balloon angio-

plasty. More detailed longer-term follow-up studies are warrented to determine the true clinical role of this emerging technology. In the future, larger expandable probes may provide adequate recanalization of peripheral lesions without the need for subsequent balloon angioplasty; sole laser thermal angioplasty may decrease the incidence of restenosis by leaving behind a smoother arterial lumen [3] than that presently observed (Fig. 5-1).

REFERENCES

1. Cumberland DC, Sanborn TA, Tayler DI, Moore DJ, Welsh CL, Greenfield AJ, Guben JK, Ryan TJ: Percutaneous laser thermal angioplasty: Initial clinical results with a laser probe in total peripheral artery occlusions. Lancet I:1457–1459, 1986.

2. Sanborn TA, Greenfield AJ, Guben JK, Menzoian JO, LoGerfo FW: Human percutaneous and intraoperative laser thermal angioplasty: Initial clinical results as an adjunct to balloon angioplasty. J Vasc Surgery 5:83–90, 1987.

3. Sanborn TA, Cumberland DC, Greenfield AJ, Welsh CL, Guben JK: Percutaneous laser thermal angioplasty: Initial results and 1-year follow-up in 129 femoropopliteal lesions. Radiology 168:121–125, 1988.

4. Sanborn TA, Faxon DP, Haudenschild C, Ryan TJ: Experimental angioplasty: Circumferential distribution of laser thermal energy with a laser probe. J Am Coll Cardiol 5:934–938, 1985.

5. Sanborn TA, Haudenschild CC, Garber GR, Ryan TJ, Faxon DP: Angiographic and histologic consequences of laser thermal angioplasty: Comparison to balloon angioplasty. Circulation 75:1281–1286, 1987.

6. Cumberland DC, Tayler DI, Procter AE: Laser-assisted percutaneous angioplasty: Initial clinical experience in peripheral arteries. Clin Radiol 37:423–428, 1986.

7. Sanborn TA, Cumberland DC, Greenfield AJ, Motarjeme A, Schwarten DE, Leachman DR, Ferris EJ, Myler RK, McCowan TC, Tatpoti D, Ginsburg R, White RI: Peripheral laser-assisted balloon angioplasty: Initial multicenter experience in 219 peripheral arteries. Arch Surg 1989.

8. Hewes RC, White RI, Murray RR, Kaufman SL, Chang R, Kadir S, Kinnison ML, Mitchell SE, Auster M: Long-term results of superficial femoral artery angioplasty. Am J Radiol 146:1025–1029, 1986.

9. Murray RR, Hewes RC, White RI, Mitchell SE, Auster M, Chang R, Kadir S, Kinnison ML, Kaufman SL: Long segment femoropopliteal stenoses: Is angioplasty a boon or a bust? Radiology 162:473–476, 1987.

10. Krepel VM, van Andel GJ, van Erp WFM, Breslaw PJ: Percutaneous transluminal angioplasty of the femoro-

popliteal artery: Initial and long-term results. Radiology 156:325–328, 1985.

11. Sos TA, Sniderman KW: Percutaneous transluminal angioplasty. Semin Roentgenol XVI:26–41, 1981.

12. Gardiner GA, Myerovitz MF, Stokes KR, Clouse ME, Harrington DP, Bettmann MA: Complications of transluminal angioplasty. Radiology 159:201–208, 1986.

13. Ginsburg R, Wexler L, Mitchell RS, Profitt D: Percutaneous transluminal laser angioplasty for treatment of peripheral vascular disease. Clinical experience with 16 patients. Radiology 156:619–624, 1985.

14. Welsh AJ, Bradley AB, Torres JH, Motamedi M, Ghidori JJ, Pearse JA, Hussein H, O'Rourke RA: Laser probe ablation of normal and atherosclerotic human aortic in vitro: A first thermographic and histologic analysis. Circulation 76:1353–1363, 1987.

6. Clinical Laser Angioplasty Experience at Northern General Hospital and the San Francisco Heart Institute

David C. Cumberland, F.R.C.R, F.R.C.P., **John R. Crew,** M.D., **Richard K. Myler,** M.D., F.A.C.C., **Simon H. Stertzer,** M.D., F.A.C.C., **Anna M. Belli,** F.R.C.R., **Robert J. Bowes,** M.R.C.P., **and Christopher L. Welsh,** F.R.C.S.

CLINICAL LASER ANGIOPLASTY EXPERIENCE

Our first experiences in laser angioplasty were in the femoral/popliteal segment using direct laser energy. [1]. A 200 or 400 μm quartz fiber connected to a continuous wave argon laser generator was passed through a 7F Teflon catheter with its tip sited either at stenoses (n = 4) or in the vessel lumen distal to occlusions (n = 11), the occlusion having been traversed by conventional guidewire/catheter methods beforehand, thus ensuring an intraluminal position of the fiber. The fiber tip was protruded 2 mm from that of the catheter. During laser-energy delivery, the catheter and fiber were held stationary in stenoses, but in occlusions they were gradually withdrawn as a combination while contrast medium was flushed to monitor progress. Lumen improvement, measured angiographically, was seen in two-thirds of the lesions, but in 2 of 11 occlusions extravasation of the contrast medium occurred, indicating perforation of the vessel wall [1]. There were no other complications, and all procedures were successfully completed with balloon dilatation. However, these instances of perforation clearly indicated the limitations of using direct laser energy with conventional delivery methods during angioplasty, bearing in mind that the fiber was known to have been intraluminal and that laser energy was given only during withdrawal of the catheter.

The thermal laser probe, with which such promising experimental results had been achieved [2], had clear practical advantages from the start: its radiopacity and provision of tactile feedback made it compatible with conventional angiographic methods. In our early experience with the laser probe, there were several device modifications, and to gain familiarity with it, we used some probes with a guidewire channel so that lesions could first be crossed with a guidewire and then the probe advanced over it. We also used the probe alone, that is without a leading guidewire, to cross some isolated stenoses as well as occlusions. A probe detachment in one of our early cases led to the provision of a "safety wire" attached to the probe, initially long enough for its proximal end to remain out of the patient, thus allowing retrieval of the tip if it detached. This design then gave way to one with a short wire with its proximal end attached to the quartz fiber, but the concept of a long wire has persisted in the "plus" design, the idea being to enable greater axial force to be used if desired and to provide some (albeit very limited) directional control of the probe.

Eventually, the optimum probe was thought to be of an olive shape of 2.0 mm diameter, mounted on a 400 μm core fiber. We soon learned that low laser powers (about 6 W or below) or keeping the probe stationary as it cools down resulted in adherence to the vessel wall. We therefore decided on the routine use of 10 W power with the 2.0 mm probe.

TECHNIQUES

The laser probe should not be regarded as a "magic bullet," the results produced being independent of case selection or technique; this will almost certainly apply to any laser-powered or other new angioplasty device. There is a definite learning curve associated with using the laser probe: the following paragraphs describe the authors' techniques and attempt to give practical "hints and wrinkles."

First, the probe should be allowed to heat up before

Laser Angioplasty, pages 35–45
© 1989 Alan R. Liss, Inc.

being applied to the obstruction. A balance has to be achieved between holding it still with laser power applied in the vessel, which probably overheats the wall [3], and excessive motion that may cool the probe too much and thus reduce its effectiveness. Our method is to hold it still just clear of the occlusion for about 2 s to allow it to heat up and then apply gentle intermittent pressure on the occlusion by moving the probe back and forth. If the probe enters the occlusion, this back-and-forth motion is continued as the probe edges forward. The laser power is discontinued either when the probe has successfully entered the patent lumen beyond the occlusion or after a (somewhat arbitrary) period of 20 s.[1] As the probe cools it is important to keep it moving for a few seconds by a rapid to-and-fro motion to avoid its sticking to the artery wall—adherence should not be a problem if this is routinely done. If the probe does stick to the wall, it can be freed by heating it up again and withdrawing it. If power is discontinued while the probe is within the occlusion, then it is often worth trying to gently advance it without laser power applied: sometimes a previously resistant portion of the occlusion will yield, possibly because it has been "softened up."

Occasionally, the probe will cross a lesion entirely when cold, but this is rare, and usually it will only advance a short distance—power then has to be applied and the back-and-forth motion with gentle forward pressure repeated. If the probe meets a particularly resistant portion of the occlusion, we abut the probe on to it with slightly increasing pressure for longer periods, progressing to moderate pressure (but never force) with the probe held still for about 3 s. If it does not go then, in our experience, it is very unlikely that it will do so, and the application of much pressure and/or prolonged heat in one place is more likely to result in wall entry or perforation than in success. This applies particularly in the adductor canal and in the popliteal artery, where perforations are more likely. Also, if the probe buckles and looks as if it would advance at an angle if allowed to, then pressure should be stopped. This is particularly likely to happen in iliac occlusions, probably partly because of the greater vessel diameter and, therefore, room for it to do so, and possibly also because some iliac occlusions are very resistant.

If the probe is not performing well, it is worth taking it out and checking whether an insulating coat of charred tissue or clot has formed on its surface. If so, scraping

this coat away with the blunt edge of a scalpel blade and wiping it firmly with swabs should clean it; this may transform the probe's effectiveness.

The "flex" probe, that is the one without the accompanying long wire, can follow vessel anatomy and curvature to a degree, but lacks "pushability." If axial support to the fiber is thought desirable, the "plus" probe, with its attached but otherwise separate wire, can be tried, but again force should not be used. The direction of the plus probe can be altered a little by pulling on either the fiber or the wire: this can be useful if there is a proximal collateral that the probe persistently enters or to aid passage within an occlusion. Control is, however, very limited, and this is an aspect under investigation.

A smaller probe, for example, one of 1.5 mm diameter instead of 2.00 mm, will get hotter for a given laser power setting and presents a lower mechanical profile. This can therefore be tried if the 2 mm probe fails, though we have not had much experience with it. We prefer to remove the 2 mm probe in the event of failure and revert to conventional angioplasty methods with a straight guidewire and curved catheter to give support and directional control [4]. Some occlusions can be treated by a combination of conventional and laser-probe methods, switching from one to the other in different sections of the occlusion if difficulty is experienced: conventional methods and the laser probe should not be regarded as mutually exclusive. For example, in common iliac occlusions, the probe may successfully negotiate most of the lesion but be unable to take the necessary curve to enter the aortic lumen at the proximal end; in this situation, pressure must not be applied. The task may be completed by changing to a curved catheter and a leading guidewire. Another example is when the probe has entered the vessel wall; this situation may be retrievable by negotiating at the point where the false channel is thought to have started, again using a straight wire supported by a curved catheter [4].

If the probe has passed successfully through the occlusion and its intraluminal position verified angiographically, it is almost always necessary (except sometimes in the tibial arteries) to produce a definitive lumen by balloon dilatation (Fig. 6–1). The quartz fiber can be cut proximally and the balloon catheter advanced over it, the fiber thus acting as a guidewire: this has the advantage of adhering to the time-honored angiographic principle that "once you are where you wanted to be you should stay there until you've finished." If the probe is removed before balloon dilatation, the previously occluded segment has to be recrossed with a guidewire—occasionally this is unsuccessful, which is, of course, very frustrating. On the other hand, the quartz fiber

---

[1] Editor's note: Based on more recent experimental studies and clinical results in smaller tibial and coronary arteries, I currently use shorter pulses of 3–5 s to limit thermal damage (see chap 4).

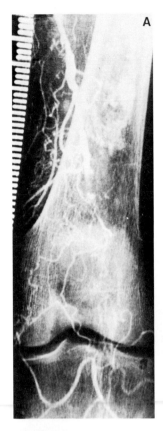
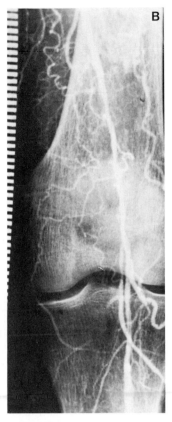
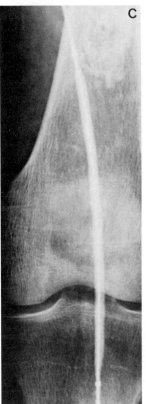
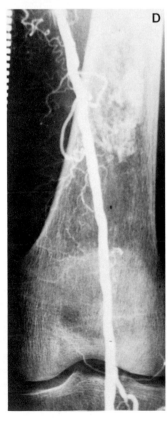

does not give very good support to the balloon catheter if the occlusion is resistant to catheter passage and it may buckle. Our practice, therefore, is to remove the probe and then very carefully negotiate the recently recanalized segment with a floppy-tipped guidewire.

A possible further advantage of removing the probe *before* balloon dilatation is to do so with power applied so as to "debulk" the occluding material as much as possible: there is some evidence that patency rates are improved by the combination of laser-probe use and balloon dilatation (see chap. 10); this may be due to such partial ablation of the occluding material or to modification of the response of the artery wall to balloon dilatation. Interestingly, many investigators using the laser probe have separately and spontaneously commented upon the unusually smooth final appearance of the vessel (Fig. 6–1), contrasting with the prominent clefts and residual filling defects commonly seen when balloon dilatation alone is used in peripheral angioplasty, particularly of occlusions and diffuse disease; clearly, a randomized trial will be necessary to confirm any benefit in terms of long-term patency. When withdrawing the probe we always do so gradually, accompanied by to-and-fro movement, with laser power applied. Usually there is definite further luminal clearance; if not, we find it helpful to check the probe's surface for adherent clot or tissue and to clean it up prior to reintroduction if significant coating has been found.

The optimum drug treatment is not known, and, as in angioplasty as a whole, there are variations in drug regimens between centers. We have not changed our drug treatment in peripheral angioplasty since using the laser probe because we have not seen any undue incidence of acute thromboembolic complications or reocclusions with its use, except possibly when the tibial arteries are subjected to much manipulation. Our policy is to give aspirin 75 mg daily unless there is contraindication, in which case dipyridamole 100 mg t.d.s. are used. If possible, these are started at least 1 day before the procedure and continued indefinitely thereafter. During the procedures, 3,000–5,000 U of heparin are given intraarterially; heparin is not continued afterward except after recanalization of long occlusions associated with poor runoff or after extensive manipulation in the

Fig. 6–1. **A,** 9 cm occlusion of left popliteal artery, not traversable with guidewire despite sustained attempts. **B,** The 2 mm thermal laser probe using 10 W of laser power has traversed the lesion producing a moderate luminal channel. **C,** Balloon dilatation. **D,** Definitive lumen produced by balloon dilatation. Good clinical result maintained, follow-up 3 years. Reproduced with permission of D.C. Cumberland et al. (Lancet 1:1457–1459, 1986).

tibial arteries; in these cases, heparinization is continued for 24 h. Before the below-knee vessels are instrumented, either with guidewires or the laser probe, 100–400 µg of glyceryl trinitrate is always given intraarterially: tibial spasm is particularly likely in women.

RESULTS WITH THE THERMAL LASER PROBE

Our experience in femoral/popliteal stenoses, gained early on while we were becoming familiar with the probe, can be quickly summarized: Of 22 stenoses, including some very eccentric lesions, all were crossed successfully with the probe alone, resulting in improvement in the mean minimum lumen diameter measured angiographically (i.e., smallest measured lumen diameter at the lesion site) from 0.75 mm ± 0.38 (SD) to 1.72 mm ± 0.52. Subsequent balloon dilatation, performed in all, provided a mean minimum lumen diameter of 3.19 mm ± 0.85. There were no complications or acute occlusions in the early postprocedure period.

Of greater interest is the ability of the probe to cross complete occlusions, particularly those lesions that could not be traversed, despite definitive attempts, by conventional means (Fig. 6–1). We initially categorized such occlusions as probably "easy" or "difficult" to cross by guidewire/catheter methods [5] and as "impossible" if either a previous sustained attempt had failed or if angioplasty would not have been attempted had the probe not been available (e.g., chronic popliteal occlusions extending into the tibial arteries [5]). More recently, we have grouped the "easy" and "difficult" categories, which are necessarily subjective in definition, as "possible," that is occlusions potentially amenable to conventional angioplasty, in which a primary success rate of 75–80% would be expected [6,7]. Success is defined here as the production of a luminal channel through the obstruction by the probe *and* subsequent successful balloon dilatation; that is, less than 50% residual diameter reduction. Overall, success was achieved in 114 of 154 total peripheral artery occlusions (74%). Of 145 femoral/popliteal occlusions ranging from 1.0 to 35 cm (mean 9 cm) long, the success rate was 73%; in 84 conventionally "possible" lesions (85%), and in 61 impossible occlusions (57%), 10 of the latter being chronic occlusions extending into the tibial artery origins. Of seven iliac occlusions between 4 and 7 cm long, four were successfully recanalized and dilated (Fig. 6–2). Perforation occurred in six (4%) of all procedures, and entry into the vessel wall in a further six (4%), none with clinical sequelae. There was one instance of popliteal embolus that was not present after probe passage

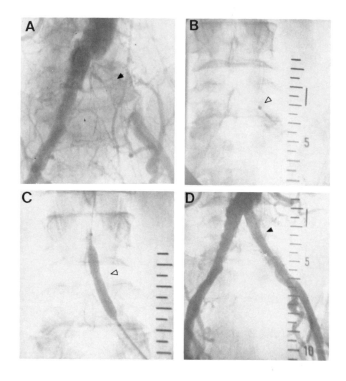

Fig. 6–2.   **A,** Left common iliac occlusion causing longstanding intermittent claudication, not traversable with guidewire. **B,** 2.5 mm Spectraprobe (arrow) traversed the lesion up to the aortic bifurcation, making guidewire/catheter passage possible. **C,** Balloon dilatation. The systolic pressure gradient of 60 mm Hg was abolished. **D,** Final angiographic result.

but occurred after subsequent balloon dilatation; this was successfully treated by percutaneous catheter suction. Acute thrombosis was observed in four patients within the first 24 h. In one further patient, cyanosis of a toe developed a few hours after a procedure, presumably due to thromboembolus from the dilated site; this resolved spontaneously.

SPECIAL TECHNIQUES AND "VARIATIONS ON THE THEME"

Debulking of Disease by 2.5-mm "Over-the-Wire" Probe

As mentioned above, debulking of the occluding material before balloon dilatation may well be beneficial, whether it be atheroma or thrombus. This may apply to stenoses, particularly diffuse disease, which can almost always be crossed with a guidewire as well as total occlusions. A 2.5 mm diameter laser probe has therefore been developed with a channel to allow its introduction over a guidewire of up to 0.035 in. diameter. This channel is eccentrically placed, enabling the probe to be rotated around the wire as it is advanced and passed back and forth through the lesion with laser power applied; this can increase the size of lumen produced, in some cases to a diameter significantly greater than 2.5 mm (Fig. 6–3). We have used this device prior to balloon dilatation in 32 stenosed femoropopliteal segments longer than 3 cm, in which there is known to be a higher recurrence rate than in shorter lesions [8], using 12 W of laser power. There have been no acute complications or early reocclusions, but it is too early to say whether long-term patency is affected. We have also used this probe in the tibial arteries, usually again followed by balloon dilatation, but in some vessels an angiographically definitive lumen has been achieved by the probe alone (Fig. 6–4). There is a peripheral laser-probe catheter of 2.5 mm diameter with a central 0.035 in. guidewire channel; as with the 2.5 mm eccentric probe, we have some as yet anecdotal experience in the tibial arteries with this device. We have been concerned about isolated instances of acute thrombosis and reocclusion in the tibial vessels with both these devices, either with or without accompanying balloon dilatation. This may be due to the nature of the disease in the vessels we have treated, sometimes being diffuse and associated with other lesions, but at the present time we are uncertain about the laser probe's role in the tibial arteries; this particularly applies to tibial stenoses, in which, with the advent of coronary angioplasty-derived materials, angioplasty has become well accepted. Certainly there is a case for continued heparinization for at least 24 h after the procedure when the probe has been used in the tibial vessels.

"Glazing"

It is well known that balloon dilatation leaves a fractured and ragged surface that is very attractive to platelets. This may be the starting point not only for acute thrombosis if either flow or blood pressure is inadequate, but also for eventual restenosis. This had led to the concept, advanced by Dr. Richard Myler, of "Glasing" the inner surface of the vessel by using the laser

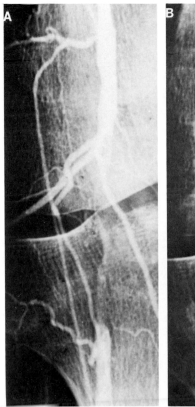
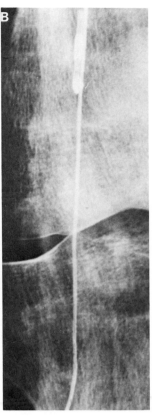
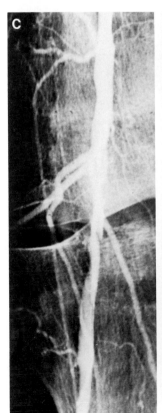
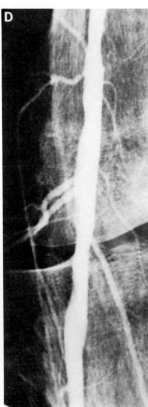

Fig. 6–3. **A,** Very severe stenosis of the popliteal artery, which is almost occluded. **B,** This lesion was easily crossed with a 0.035 in. guidewire. Over this guidewire, a 2.5 mm thermal laser probe with an eccentric guidewire channel was repeatedly passed through the diseased segment using 12 W of laser power. **C,** After this "debulking" maneuver, there is significant lumen improvement. **D,** Final lumen after balloon dilatation showing definitive, smooth lumen.

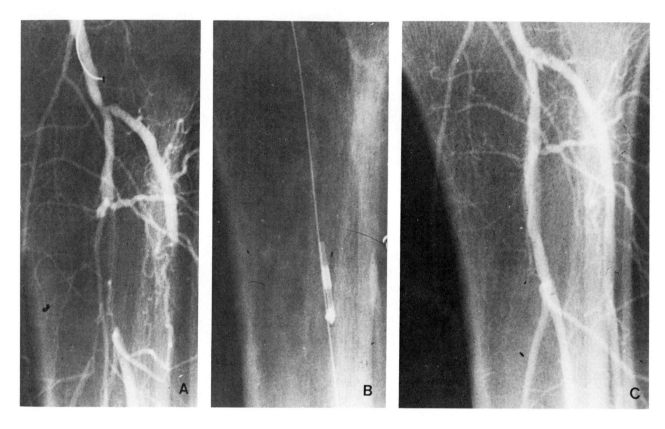

Fig. 6–4. **A,** Angiogram of the distal end of the popliteal artery and its branches showing very severe stenosis of the posterior tibial artery, occlusion of the anterior tibial artery several centimeters after its origin, and stenosis at the anterior tibial origin. **B,** The posterior tibial stenosis was crossed with a 0.014 in. steerable guidewire over which a 2.5 mm eccentric laser probe was introduced. Using 12 W of laser power, the probe was repeatedly passed through the posterior tibial stenosis. **C,** Definitive lumen produced by the laser probe. The occlusion of the anterior tibial artery and the stenosis at its origin were treated by conventional balloon dilatation.

probe *after* balloon dilatation. This can be done with an over-the-wire probe using the same guidewire as the one used for the balloon catheter. The probe is moved back and forth across the dilated area several times during applications of laser power. This maneuver does appear to be safe; from our experience of 34 femoral/popliteal segments, we have not observed any complications or deterioration in the angiographic appearances. In 12 of these cases, there has been some angiographic improvement (Fig. 6–5), usually taking

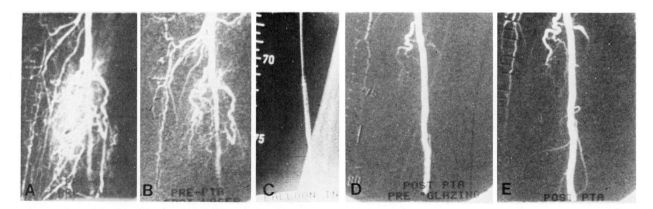

Fig. 6–5. **A,B:** Digital angiograms of a 5 cm left superficial femoral occlusion with a severe stenosis about 2 cm distally. These lesions were crossed with a 2.0 mm thermal laser probe and then balloon dilated (**C**). **D,** After dilatation, there is a generally good lumen, but at the site of the previous severe distal stenosis, there is clearly a defect and possible intimal cleft. The laser probe was then repeatedly passed up and down this segment using 10 W of laser power, providing definite angiographic improvement (**E**).

the form of reduction in filling defects, but sometimes in apparent lessening of residual stenosis. Some angioscopic support for the glazing concept has been obtained intraoperatively [9]. As with "debulking" prior to balloon dilatation, whether acute reocclusion or recurrence can be reduced by glazing is not known, and a randomized trial will not be appropriate until some knowledge of the optimum method can be gained by either animal experiments or detailed angioscopic observations. For example, whether high or low laser power should be used is a matter of current debate.

Alternative Approaches

Percutaneous use of the laser probe requires an arterial sheath, precluding its use for lesions near the inguinal ligament. There are several alternatives: 1) open arteriotomy, 2) the introduction of the probe from a distant site such as the contralateral groin, and 3) the popliteal approach.

Open arteriotomy. This is useful when there is common femoral disease that precludes local catheter-

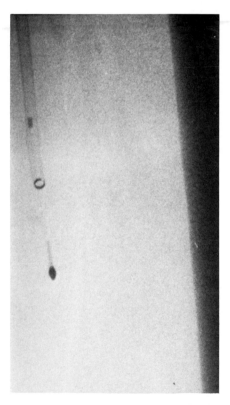

Fig. 6–6. Frame from cineangiographic film showing 9 F giant lumen Interventional Medical guiding catheter, introduced from the opposite femoral artery, guiding a 2.0 mm probe in a superficial femoral artery occlusion.

ization and that requires surgical clearance at the same time as angioplasty of proximal or distal lesions. We have also often performed open procedures when the superficial femoral artery is occluded at its origin.

The contralateral or "crossover" approach. At the time of writing, a 9 F coronary angioplasty guiding catheter with an inner lumen capable of carrying a 2.0 mm laser probe (Interventional Medical Inc.) has just become available (Fig. 6–6). With the aid of a guidewire, we have passed the right coronary version of this guiding catheter over the aortic bifurcation and distally until it lies about 2 cm proximal to the occlusion point. The tip shape and torque characteristics of the catheter allow some directional control of the probe, and we are investigating the role of this combination in common femoral and superficial femoral origin occlusions. This is hopefully a prelude to selective laser-assisted angioplasty of such vessels as the renal, mesenteric and upper limb arteries.

The popliteal approach. This method has been used for superficial femoral artery occlusions starting at the vessel origin, which are very difficult to enter from above [10]. As mentioned above, the laser probe at present has very limited steerability. Collaterals proximal to an occlusion may be persistently entered, particularly if there is only a gradual angle with the parent vessel and if a stump at the occlusion point cannot be identified. Screening in different oblique projections may reveal such a stump, but even so, failure to enter the occlusion can result. Indeed, some instances of perforation may well be due to undetected entry into a small collateral vessel, the probe then perforating the collateral if force is used. By contrast, the distal end of occlusions is usually symmetrical and concave, presenting a favorable configuration for entry from below. Such femoral occlusions can be approached by catheterizing the popliteal artery. Guidance for the percutaneous puncture of the vessel is provided by prior cannulation of the common femoral artery and injections of contrast medium while the puncture is made under fluoroscopic control with the patient prone. The angioplasty then proceeds as with an antegrade approach, though particular care both during and after the procedure is necessary to avoid a hematoma. We have not yet had enough experience with this technique to judge whether it could be a frequent alternative to the proximal antegrade approach.

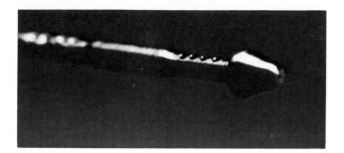

Fig. 6–7. The 2.5-mm Spectraprobe.

The Spectraprobe

The Spectraprobe™ has a window at its tip with a recessed sapphire lens (Fig. 6–7); depending on the design, this allows a proportion of the input laser energy to pass through the lens and thus to interact directly with tissue. In the design we have used, about 18% of the energy is so transmitted and the remainder is absorbed by the probe to be converted into heat. The possible advantages of this "hybrid" probe with a combination of laser/thermal effect were first put forward by Abela et al. [11]. They suggested that the direct energy provided a "pilot channel" for the probe to follow, a notion that has since been supported by further experiments [12].

We have used a 2.5 mm Spectraprobe with 12 W input energy, usually argon wavelength but recently using an Nd-YAG generator, in 34 total peripheral artery occlusions, 10 iliac and 24 femoral/popliteal/tibial,

with 79% success; there have been one perforation and four instances of vessel wall entry, none with sequelae. These crude figures tend to belie our impression that the Spectraprobe does indeed cross occlusions more rapidly and quickly than the 2.0 mm entirely thermal probe, with which we have more experience. It is also noteworthy that the mean minimum lumen diameter produced by the 2.5 mm Spectraprobe is larger relative to its own diameter than that provided by the 2.0 mm thermal probe, being 2.44 ± .078 mm compared with 1.34 ± 0.29 mm (Fig. 6–8). On the other hand, it is difficult to be sure that these apparent advantages are due to the window and the partially direct laser effect: the Spectraprobe has a slightly different configuration and has a stiffer 600 μm core fiber compared with the 400 μm fiber of the 2.0 mm probe; also, we have found that the window usually becomes obscured by clot and/or tissue at some stage during the procedure.

The "Laserwire"

This device is basically a 0.018 in. diameter thermal laser probe, with the outward appearance and to some extent the handling characteristics of a steerable guide wire. With only 3–3.5 W of input laser energy, the tip will reach a temperature of 1,000°C. We have used the device in several complete tibial artery occlusions that were too resistant for conventional small-bore guidewires, with some success (Fig. 6–9). At the time of writing, we have been assessing its role in percutaneous angioplasty of total coronary occlusions (see chap. 11).

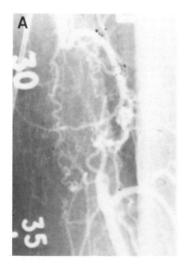
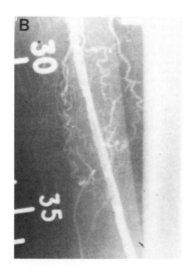
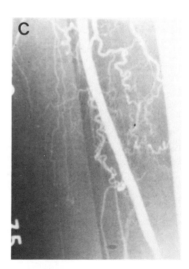

Fig. 6–8. Short left superficial femoral occlusion. **B,** After the occlusion has been traversed with a 2.5 mm Spectraprobe using 12 W of laser power, a good, but not quite definitive, lumen has been produced. **C,** After balloon dilatation showing definitive lumen.

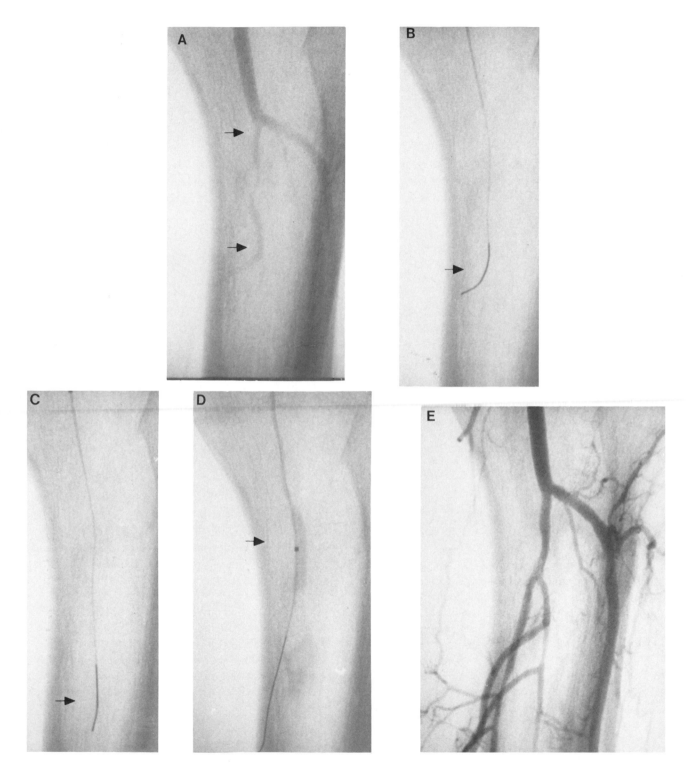

Fig. 6–9. **A,** Angiogram of the distal portion of the left popliteal artery and its branches. Severe stenosis (bounded by arrows) of the common peroneal artery. Distally, the superficial peroneal artery is occluded. **B,** The 0.018 in. laser wire with an eccentric tip, using 3.0 W of laser power, was used to traverse the common peroneal stenosis and distally entered a peroneal branch. **C,** There was sufficient torque control to steer the wire out of the peroneal branch, and, again using laser power, the peroneal occlusion was traversed. **D,** Balloon dilatation of the common peroneal stenosis. The previously occluded superficial peroneal segment was also balloon dilated, as was a stenosis near the origin of the deep peroneal (posterior tibial) artery revealed during fluoroscopy. **E,** Final angiographic result.

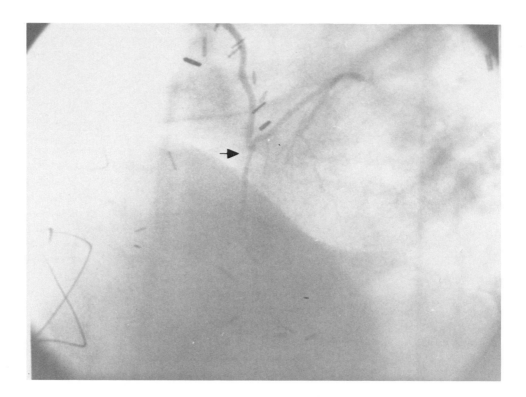

Fig. 6–10.   Follow-up angiogram of an IMA to LAD laser weld. Left anterior oblique (LAO) 60°, cranial (CR) 15° projection, 1 week post left internal mammary artery–left anterior descending (LIMA-LAD) bypass graft in a 72-year-old man. Laser welding was used for the anastomosis (arrow). (Figure courtesy of John Crew, M.D., Seton Medical Center, Daly City, CA.)

Direct Laser Catheter

Early experiences using direct laser energy with conventional fibers and machines were mentioned at the beginning of this chapter. There has been much research into improving delivery methods for direct laser-assisted angioplasty. One of us (S.H.S.) has been involved in the development of a catheter with multiple fibers through which high-powered short pulses of argon energy are delivered, providing histologically precise, well-defined channels. After preliminary use in peripheral vessels, this catheter is now being assessed in the coronary arteries (see chap. 11).

Laser Welding

Following successful experimental use of low-energy direct argon laser welding in a canine model [13], we have used this technique to repair human brachial arteriotomies following cardiac interventional procedures [14]. This method has the potential advantages of allowing healing of vessel wall intima, media and adventitia without the foreign body reaction secondary to sutures, of restoring normal capacitance without suture (purse string) restraint, and of allowing opportunity for normal tissue growth without scarring or compromised luminal diameter or blood flow. In 20 human brachial arteries repaired with low-energy direct argon laser welding, there were no significant complications or evidence of luminal narrowing over a 2-month follow-up. The technique has now been extended to the intraoperative coronary setting (Fig. 6–10).

THE FUTURE

Definitive lumen production by laser/thermal means alone is presently possible in some tibial arteries and very occasionally in the femoral/popliteal segments. Hotter probes, expandable ones, or even multiple probes alongside each other are being investigated to achieve this goal, which appears from animal experiments to be a desirable one [15]. Suggested advantages, discussed above, of either debulking or glazing in cooperation with balloon dilatation, or obviating the need for the mechanical injury of balloon dilatation altogether, remain to be proven in clinical practice.

Larger lumen guiding catheters are allowing large or multiple devices to be passed down them—this may become relevant to angioplasty of vessels requiring selective catheterization, including the coronary arteries.

The Spectraprobe, even with the caveats mentioned above, is a promising device. There will be variations in design, such as in probe shape and in the size and position of the window; also new wavelengths and delivery systems may be used to provide different combinations of laser/thermal tissue interaction.

We have shown that the laser wire will cross some total occlusions of the tibial and coronary arteries that were hitherto inaccessible (Fig. 6–9 and chap. 11). Further experience will determine to what extent the applicability of angioplasty will thus be increased.

The peripheral vessels, an important area for treatment and for technical advancement in their own right, will no doubt remain the testing ground for new devices, even for those whose ultimate goal is the coronary arteries. The team approach, practiced in our institutions, in which cardiologist, radiologist, and surgeon work together, has broadened our scope and increased our treatment possibilities; we believe that this is the best way to advance the cause of angioplasty.

ACKNOWLEDGMENTS

We should like to thank Benito Hidalgo, R.T., and Marilyn Dean, R.V.T., for their invaluable technical assistance.

REFERENCES

1. Cumberland DC, Tayler DI, Procter AE: Laser-assisted percutaneous angioplasty—Initial clinical experience in the peripheral arteries. Clin Radiol 37:423–428, 1986.

2. Sanborn TA, Faxon DP, Haudenschild CC, Ryan TJ: Experimental angioplasty: Circumferential distribution of laser thermal energy with a laser probe. J Am Coll Cardiol 5:934–938, 1984.

3. Welch AJ, Bradley AB, Torres JH, Motamedi M, Ghidoni JJ, Pearce JA, Hussein H, O'Rourke RA: Laser probe ablation of normal and atherosclerotic human aorta in vitro: A first thermographic and histologic analysis. Circulation 76:1353–1363, 1987.

4. Carver RA, Cumberland DC: Use of a cobra-shaped catheter to effect recanalisation of femoro-popliteal occlusions. J Intervent Radiol 2:97–98, 1987.

5. Cumberland DC, Sanborn TA, Tayler DI, Moore DJ, Welsh CL, Greenfield AJ, Guben JK, Ryan TJ: Percutaneous laser thermal angioplasty: Initial clinical results with a laser probe in total peripheral artery occlusions. Lancet 1:1457–1459, 1986.

6. Zeitler E, Richter EI, Sayferth W: Femoro-popliteal arteries. In Dotter CR, Gruentzig AR, Schoop W, Zeitler E (eds): Percutaneous Transluminal Angioplasty. Technique, Early and Late Results. Berlin: Springer-Verlag, 1983:105–114.

7. Cumberland DC: Present status of angioplasty. In Sherwood T, Steiner RE (eds): Recent Advances in Radiology and Medical Imaging. Edinburgh: Churchill Livingstone, 1986:165–185.

8. Gallino A, Mahler F, Probst P, Nachbur B: Percutaneous transluminal angioplasty of the arteries of the lower limbs: A 5 year follow-up. Circulation 70:619–623, 1984.

9. Myler RK, Cumberland DA, Clark DA, Stertzer SH, Tatpati DA, Sen Sarma PK: High and low energy thermal laser angioplasty for total occlusions and restenosis in man (abstract). Circulation 76:IV–230, 1987.

10. Siragusa V, Bowers JA, Thomas HM: Laser angioplasty of totally occluded superficial femoral arteries via a percutaneous popliteal approach. Journal of Interventional Cardiology 1:199–207, 1988.

11. Abela GS, Seeger JM, Barbieri E, Franzini D, Fenech A, Pepine CJ, Conti CR: Laser angioplasty with angioscopic guidance in humans. J Am Coll Cardiol 8:184–192, 1986.

12. Yang Y, Hashizume M, Arbutina D, Milewski LF, DuPree J, Matsumoto T: Argon laser angioplasty with a laser probe. J Vasc Surg 60:60–65, 1987.

13. White RA, Kopchok G, Donayre C, White G, Lyons R, Fujitani R, Klein SR, Uitto J: Argon laser welded arteriovenous anastomoses. J Vasc Surg 6:447–454, 1987.

14. Crew JR, Stertzer SH, Myler RK, Clark DC, White R, Dean M: Blood vessel welding by laser: Use of photochemical covalent bonding in clinical application (abstract). Circulation 76:IV–230, 1987.

15. Sanborn TA, Haudenschild CC, Garber GR, Ryan TJ, Faxon DP: Angiographic and histologic consequences of laser thermal angioplasty: Comparison with balloon angioplasty. Circulation 75:1281–1286, 1987.

7. Laser Recanalization: The Hybrid Probe

Gérald Barbeau, M.D., **George S. Abela**, M.D., and **James M. Seeger**, M.D.

INTRODUCTION

The advent of balloon angioplasty has opened the way for consideration of other percutaneous recanalization techniques. Laser and laser thermal recanalization procedures were among the first to be evaluated. One advantage of the laser is the ability to vaporize tissue both in a selective and a precise fashion [1–3]. Since the laser leaves behind a relatively smooth surface when compared to balloon angioplasty, it has the potential for less restenosis and sudden occlusion [4–6]. The laser also has the potential of treating arteries that are diffusely narrowed or totally occluded. Such vessels usually are not considered to be treatable with conventional revascularization procedures such as bypass surgery or balloon angioplasty. A final advantage of laser recanalization is that, as a percutaneous procedure, it can be repeated on numerous occasions, thus postponing the need for bypass surgery. Laser recanalization may provide yet another alternative therapy to bypass surgery and balloon angioplasty for the treatment of arterial obstructions.

CARDIOVASCULAR LASER STUDIES

Early In Vitro Experimental Studies

Preliminary work evaluating the direct effect of lasers on arterial tissue demonstrated that laser impact on atherosclerotic plaque created a central zone of vaporization surrounded by a secondary zone of thermal coagulation and, frequently, a third zone of acoustic shock trauma [1]. Thus, plaque could be successfully reduced into its elemental components, namely, water vapor, carbon dioxide, and other aromatic combustion by-products [7]. It is, however, the availability of small flexible optical fibers that allows the adaptation of laser techniques for percutaneous angioplasty procedures. Since laser angioplasty is performed in an enclosed space, namely, the vascular lumen, the interaction between the laser and arterial tissue is greatly influenced by the interceding medium. Early predictions suggested that laser delivery through a blood-filled vessel would not vaporize plaque effectively. Experimental results, however, have proven that laser recanalization can be effectively performed in both saline or whole blood medium with minimal hemolysis and debris formation [8–10].

In Vivo Technical Problems

Early experiments, conducted in animal models, were done mainly in the peripheral circulation of atherosclerotic rabbits. These studies demonstrated the feasibility of laser recanalization in stenosed or occluded arterial segments; however, the perforation rate was high and channel size was limited to the size of the diameter of the fiber [11]. Studies where the bare fiber was used with or without fluoroscopic guidance resulted in a very high (90%) perforation rate. This was also associated with backburning of the tip of the optical fiber. The fiber core melted following contact with the atheromatous plaque. Two factors appeared to influence perforation rate. These were the mechanical and optical behavior of the bare optical fiber. In order to reduce the perforation rate and to enhance the channel diameter size, several modifications were introduced into the tip of the optical fiber as well as in the guiding system.

Fluoroscopic Guidance and Catheter Systems

Since the optical fiber is radiolucent, the tip of the bare fiber could not be seen by fluoroscopy. In order to resolve this problem, a metallic ring was inserted on the tip of the optical fiber to make it radiopaque and allow fluoroscopic visualization. Subsequently, the fiber was placed through a guiding angiographic catheter and protruded during recanalization from the end of the catheter [12]. An unanticipated advantage of the metal ring at the end of the fiber was that it protected the fiber tip from backburning. This prolonged the working life of the optical fiber system during the procedure and provided reliable laser delivery to the plaque. Although the perforation rate seemed somewhat reduced when using this system in straight peripheral arteries of atherosclerotic rabbits, it was obvious that advancing this system inside normal coronary arteries resulted in frequent perforations. The mechanical stiffness as well as the sharp-edged tip of the fiber continued to pose significant problems in tortuous vessels. In an experiment done in coronary arteries of live dogs, using energy levels known to recanalize atherosclerotic plaque in the rabbit model, frequent perforations resulted with consequent tamponade and death in the majority of these dogs [13].

In order to avoid mechanical perforations while advancing a stiff bare optical fiber, attempts were made to keep the fiber tip away from the arterial wall. One method was to shield the optical fiber in a catheter body and to deliver laser radiation on a pull back [14]. Another approach was to use a balloon-tipped catheter to keep the fiber centralized in the arterial lumen [15]. In spite of these approaches, perforations persisted, which were still related to the misalignment of the laser fiber and exiting beam within the coronary arteries of a beating heart.

Angioscopy

In order to improve the delivery of laser recanalization without perforation, angioscopy was evaluated as an approach to help guide the laser fiber. Angioscopy provided a clear assessment of vascular pathology including the nature as well as the exact site of the vascular obstruction [8]. Unfortunately, angioscopy did not prevent vessel perforation during laser recanalization since there was little control over the direction of the optical fiber. Additionally, the narrow field of vision ($< 40°$ full angle) and the inability to visualize the laser fiber as it advanced through an obstruction did not provide any indication of the perforation even after it occurred. Other limitations of angioscopy in these early studies were related to the bulky size of the angioscopes as well as the lack of user friendliness. This included the need for continuous saline flush in order to visualize the lumen and localize the obstruction. Subsequent improvements with current angioscopes have rekindled the interest in angioscopy as a technique for evaluation of vascular pathology during interventional procedures [16]. This is mainly related to the reduction in size of the angioscope (< 1 mm diameter), the improved flexibility, and reduced fragility.

The Laser Probe

A further modification of the metal ring at the tip of the fiber resulted in encapsulation of the tip of the optical fiber in an elliptical bullet-shaped metallic cap. This converted the delivery system into an exclusively thermal system or "laser probe" [17,18]. Several studies were performed comparing this laser-probe system with the bare optical fiber and demonstrated fewer perforations as a consequence of the atraumatic blunt tip at the end of the fiber [11]. In addition, the metal cap was available in different sizes (1–2.5 mm) that created larger luminal dimensions than the size of the fiber body. These two advantages, compared to the bare-fiber system, greatly enhanced the delivery system for the recanalization of occluded arteries. Histology seen with the laser probe suggested a common thermal mechanism for the recanalization process as compared to the bare fiber with the metal ring. However, the efficiency of tissue ablation seemed compromised with the discontinuation of the free laser beam. The preferential absorption of the argon wavelengths by the atherosclerotic plaque [19] and the enhanced effects of lasing through blood [20] were lost. The laser probe required high temperature and good mechanical contact with the target atheroma to effectively recanalize the obstructed segments. Another aspect of this thermal approach was that it made possible alternative mechanisms for heat-producing devices. These included catheters with less expensive energy sources such as microwave, electrical, and chemical [21,22].

The Sapphire Tip

Other attempts to reduce arterial perforation and to enhance recanalization were made. A rounded sapphire at the end of the optical fiber resulted in a smooth-ended fiber system that was mechanically less traumatic than was the bare fiber. This system also resulted in a reduction in the perforation rate; however, it also limited the size of the channel to that of the sapphire tip itself. The effect on plaque was a central area of vaporization at the beam focal point. With increased total energy, the sapphire tip heated up and acted as a contact device as evidenced by typical charring seen at the edges of the recanalized lumen. Using this system coupled to an Nd-Yag laser, peripheral arteries could be successfully recanalized in patients [23]. As in the case of the other described systems, subsequent balloon angioplasty was required to increase the luminal dimension in order to achieve adequate blood flow and to relieve symptoms in the peripheral extremities.

Other Recanalization Devices

Several other modifications have been proposed to prevent arterial perforation during laser recanalization. These have included other laser wavelengths such as the shorter-pulse excimer laser that provides more precise ablation and less surrounding vascular tissue damage [7,24]. Unfortunately, these systems are greatly limited by the same problems as described above, namely, a small-size channel requiring balloon angioplasty to enhance the lumen following the procedure. The use of chromophores such as tetracycline for selective enhancement of plaque atherolysis [25] has also been used but has not been successful in debulking large amounts of plaque. The use of fluorescence for plaque recognition and feedback control of plaque ablation has also been reported [26,27]. The use of these systems, however, has also been greatly limited by the loss of the plaque signal following ablation as well as by attenuation due to the blood medium. The use of real-time two-dimensional ultrasound analysis has also been attempted and is a promising method for detection of plaque thickness in the arterial lumen [28]. The technical difficulties to adapt this technology to the laser is an area of active research. Finally, the use of angioscopy as a guiding system is being reconsidered with newer versions of angioscopes. Nevertheless, at present, the standard fluoroscopic guidance and the use of a guidewire appears to be the most practical and feasible approach for laser recanalization. Several studies have used this approach and have demonstrated its simplicity and effectiveness [29,30]. Finally, the advent of the laser-balloon catheter as well as stents and atherectomy devices may provide alternative approaches to reduce the restenosis following conventional balloon angioplasty.

CLINICAL TRIALS

Preliminary Clinical Trials

Preliminary clinical trials with laser recanalization were done both in the United States and in Europe. The first clinical report was done using a bare optical fiber advanced through a centralizing balloon catheter [31]. This was performed in the peripheral circulation of a patient for limb salvage. No angiographic figures obtained after the procedure were included in this report; however, the patient was reported to have improved symptomatically. Subsequently, a similar approach was used with an Nd-Yag laser in the superficial femoral artery in three patients [32]. The limitation was mainly the small-size lumen channels. Also, the patients were reported to experience a slight discomfort and burning sensation throughout the lasing period; however, no major side effects occurred as a result of the procedure.

Larger series of patients were then reported using both the laser-probe system and more recently with the Lastac™ system, all requiring subsequent balloon angioplasty to improve lumen diameter [33–35]. The experience and development of the "hybrid" probe is described in the following section.

Hybrid-probe Development

In August 1984, the first FDA-approved clinical trial of laser recanalization in peripheral arteries was started at the University of Florida. Attempts were made to recanalize obstructed peripheral arteries using an argon laser coupled to an open-ended optical fiber with a metal sleeve at the tip. The initial approach was to penetrate the lesions with this probe and then to increase the power on the pull back through the lesion, to take advantage of the wide angle of the beam to increase the channel size. A 45° full-angle beam was used in these early attempts. This approach was not successful in enlarging the lumen diameter, and frequent perforations were seen due to the sharp edges of the optical-probe system. Further development included increasing the metal on the tip of the probe to widen the channel and make the tip blunt. The bare optical fiber was recessed behind the orifice of the metal tip. This resulted in a wider channel, but debris accumulated in the window at the probe tip and damaged the optical fiber. In order to prevent this fiber damage and as well as beam scatter from the fiber tip, a sapphire lens was inserted in the window at the probe tip. This modification prevented the accumulation of materials inside that channel. It also realigned and improved the beam profile exiting from the end of the fiber. This final configuration was referred to as the hybrid probe (i.e., combined thermal and optical effects), and the remainder of the clinical trial was conducted with this probe [8]. This probe was mounted on a 300 μm core silica fiber, and the window at the probe tip was 250 μm (Fig. 7–1). The accrued advantages of this system included the ability to modulate the laser beam and to create a track of least resistance in the obstructing lesion to subsequently advance the bulk of the metal probe. This approach resulted in an enhanced self-centering system during recanalization. Because of this enhanced optical and mechanical ability, the 2 mm probe resulted in fewer perforations as compared with the open-ended fiber with the metal collar.

An additional finding was that the channel created with this system was occasionally slightly wider than the probe itself. On histologic examination, a smooth endothelial surface covered with a very thin zone of charring and an underlying zone of thermal damage was observed (Fig. 7–2). In addition, scanning electron microscopy revealed a crescent-shaped zone of amorphous tissue consistent with thermal necrosis at the leading edge of the channel (Fig. 7–3). Recanalization of atherosclerotic and calcific plaque was feasible although

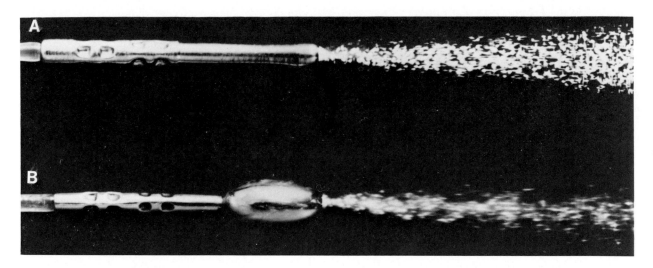

Fig. 7–1. **A,** A 300 μm core optical fiber with (A) a 1-mm metal sleeve and (**B**) a 2-mm elliptical metal sleeve at the tip. In both A and B, the back end of the sleeve is crimped onto the fiber cladding and an argon laser beam (1 W) is seen exiting from the tip at a 15° angle. The beam of the 2-mm probe in B has a narrower waist and is less intense than the 1-mm probe in A. Reproduced with permission of G.S. Abela, et al. and the American College of Cardiology (Journal of the American College of Cardiology 8:184–192, 1986).

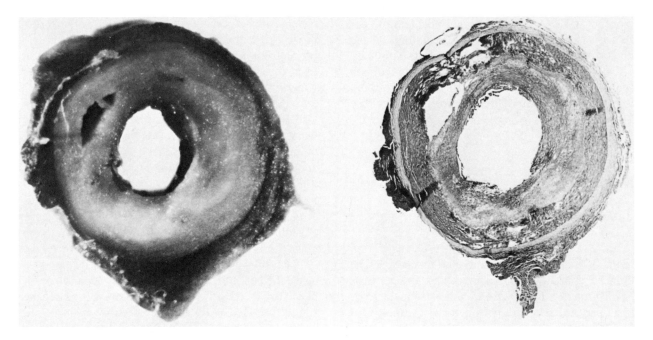

Fig. 7–2. Recanalized artery. Left: Fresh segment of superficial femoral artery after laser recanalization. The central channel was made using a 2 mm probe. The original lumen appears in the 11 o'clock position. Right: Histologic cross section of the recanalized artery illustrating relatively smooth-walled central lumen with minimal charring and thermal injury made with argon laser. The left upper quadrant shows original vascular lumen. (Hematoxylin-eosin. Magnification × 12.) Reproduced with permission of G.S. Abela et al. and the American College of Cardiology (Journal of the American College of Cardiology 8:184–192, 1986).

no sustained channel could be made in fresh thrombus. Also, very hard and heavily calcified plaque could not be effectively recanalized. A 0.016 in. flexible guidewire could be passed in an eccentric channel at the tip of the hybrid probe in a similar fashion as with the early laser-probe system. This seemed to greatly improve the alignment of the probe within the lumen of tortuous vessels. Given these modifications, it was possible to deliver both free laser beam and thermal radiation from the tip of this probe using a guidewire to align the system in the coronary artery of live dogs without perforation [29].

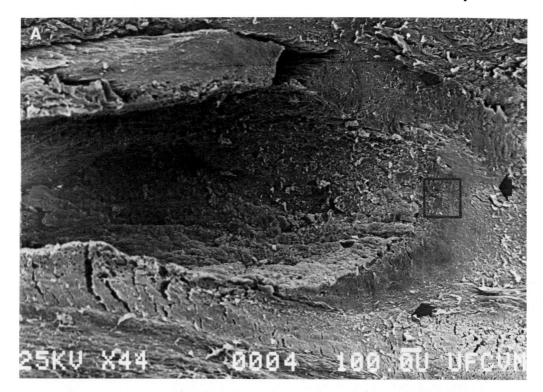

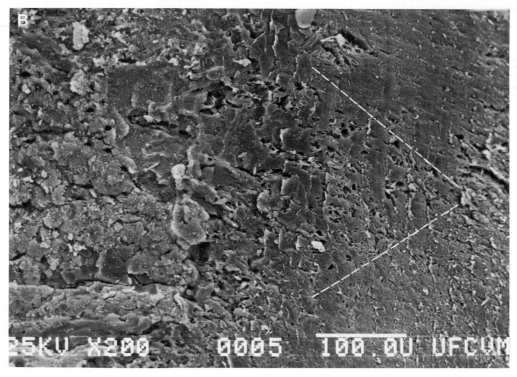

Fig. 7–3.   Scanning electron micrograph of a longitudinal section of a right superficial femoral artery. **A,** The leading edge of a newly created central vascular channel is shown. An area of crescent-shape amorphous tissue consistent with thermal necrosis is seen at the leading edge of the channel (arrows). The boxed central area of the crescent corresponds to the exiting of the laser beam and is further magnified below. White bar at bottom = 100 nm. **B,** At higher magnification, vacuolization can be seen at the center of the crescent of thermal necrosis. This is suggestive of early tissue vaporization. This area is outlined within the dotted line. White bar at bottom = 100 nm. Reproduced with permission of G.S. Abela et al. and the American College of Cardiology (Journal of the American College of Cardiology 8:184–192, 1986.)

In recent experiments comparing the efficiency of plaque ablation using both the laser-probe and hybrid-probe systems, there appeared to be more tissue volume removed with the hybrid-probe system as compared with the laser-probe system [36]. This one-to-one comparison was done under similar conditions using volumetric measurements of the ablated plaque. In addition, temperature measurement of both probes made during the experiments showed that plaque removed with the hybrid system was achieved at a lower temperature compared with the laser-probe [36].

Further Optical Modification

The major limitations of laser recanalization have been arterial perforation and the small channel size created by the currently available systems. Other approaches have involved the use of a microlens at the end of an optical fiber that provides a focused laser beam as well as a blunt and atraumatic surface. Work done at our laboratory has demonstrated that it is feasible to create a microlens at the tip of an optical fiber that results in a small angle of dispersion while maintaining a high-power density within 2 mm from the tip of the fiber [37]. This approach also reduced the amount of beam scattering commonly seen with a bare optical fiber. Such beam scattering can result in unpredictable zones of high-power density or hot spots that lead to perforation.

The effect of a microlens or sapphire lens was a realignment of the beam that resulted in more effective impact on plaque. As the lens was moved away from the plaque, there was a rapid increase in the power density as the focal point (400–500 μm from the surface of the lens) was approached. Using an argon laser beam, a bare fiber was compared to the microlens-tipped fiber in a perpendicular fashion to aortic tissue. The beam from the microlens-tipped fiber could be focused at a short distance from the tip and then dispersed. This prevented deep vessel damage and resulted in wider and shallower craters at the surface of the tissue [37]. Another advantage was that if the fiber was placed on its side and parallel to the tissue surface no lateral damage occurred even when the lens was in contact with the tissue.

The Current Hybrid Probe

The catheter currently used in our studies is the final embodiment of the hybrid-probe system. This is a commercially available system known as the Spectraprobe-PLR™ (Trimedyne, Inc., Santa Ana, CA) and is avail-

TABLE 7–1. Distribution of 60 Procedures (56 Patients), per Phase

Phase	Technical success/ procedure (%)	Perforations
1 (intraoperative)	7/9 (78)	2
2 (intraoperative)	8/13 (62)	4
3 (intraoperative)	3/6 (50)	2
3 (percutaneous)	26/32 (81)	5

Phase 1: August 1984–September 1985; phases 2 and 3: March 1986–March 1988.

able as a 2.0 or a 2.5 mm probe. These systems are mounted on either a 300- or 600-μm-core silica fiber, respectively. Approximately 15–20% of the input laser beam is allowed to escape from the tip of the probe. Additionally, there is an eccentric channel allowing for the passage of a 0.016 in. steerable guidewire that acts as a "monorail" system. All this apparatus is assembled in a 7 F thin-walled catheter to allow simultaneous contrast injection during laser recanalization.[1]

University of Florida Clinical Experience

The clinical experience with the hybrid probe was divided in three clinical phases. Phase 1 was designed as a pilot study to evaluate the immediate effects of laser recanalization. During this phase, the hybrid probe evolved from a simple fiber with a collar at the tip into the more sophisticated metal tip with a recessed sapphire lens. The initial procedures were performed intraoperatively on patients preselected to undergo peripheral bypass surgery. In phase 1, no attempt was made to recanalize the obstructed segment entirely. Following recanalization, the arterial segment was excised and microscopic and physiologic evaluation were done. During phase 2 of the study, all procedures were performed intraoperatively with the intention to do a complete revascularization. If the lumen diameter achieved was < 50% of the normal artery, then a bypass was performed. Access for the laser was via a femoral cutdown under local epidural anesthesia. In phase 3 of the study, the majority of the procedures were done via a percutaneous approach. The intraoperative cutdown was reserved for patients who could not be accessed percutaneously (Table 7–1).

Patient selection. Phase 1 extended over 1 year

---

[1]Editor's note: Other investigators in this volume describe the use of the Spectraprobe without the 7 F catheter. This catheter may offer the advantage of providing access to the distal vessel after recanalization for safe guidewire and balloon catheter exchange.

(August 1984–September 1985) and consisted of 11 patients selected for laser recanalization during bypass surgery. The hybrid probe was used in seven of these patients for nine procedures. Phases 2 and 3 were conducted between March 1986 and March 1988. During this period, 234 patients were screened as possible candidates for laser recanalization. Following an initial interview with our nurse coordinator, the patient was evaluated by either the cardiologist or vascular surgeon for clinical history and physical examination. Ischemic symptoms at rest with or without tissue loss or progressive intermittent claudication < 2 blocks were considered as clinical inclusion criteria. Occasionally, a patient with claudication > 2 blocks was considered for peripheral revascularization if the symptoms were interfering greatly with life style.

Further investigation, obtained by noninvasive examination, included segmental Doppler pressures at rest and following exercise testing, for localization and documentation of the severity of the peripheral arterial disease. Ankle brachial systolic pressure ratios were obtained before and after intervention.

When the superficial femoral or popliteal artery pressure gradients were confirmed by noninvasive technique and when a recent (< 6 months) good-quality angiogram was not available, a complete abdominal aortic angiogram and runoff was performed. Disease locations considered to be treatable included the common iliac artery, superficial femoral artery, popliteal artery, and common peroneal artery. Also, patients considered for limb salvage with severe distal tibial artery occlusions were accepted for the procedure. Presence of calcium or lesion length were not criteria for exclusion.

The patient was offered the possibility of laser recanalization after review of the history and angiogram by the radiologist, the cardiologist, and the vascular surgeon involved in the case. Of the 234 patients screened, 46 were excluded following interview with our nurse coordinator, 50 following clinical investigation, and 89 on the absence of the anatomic criteria already mentioned. An informed consent including the potential benefits and risks of the procedure was obtained. The patient was started on enteric coated aspirin 325 mg p.o. and was premedicated on the day of the procedure with Valium 10 mg p.o. and Dilaudid 2 mg im.

Laser recanalization. The percutaneous approach was performed under local anesthesia (2% lidocaine) with an arterial access obtained using a 20-gauge beveled needle directed in an antegrade fashion in

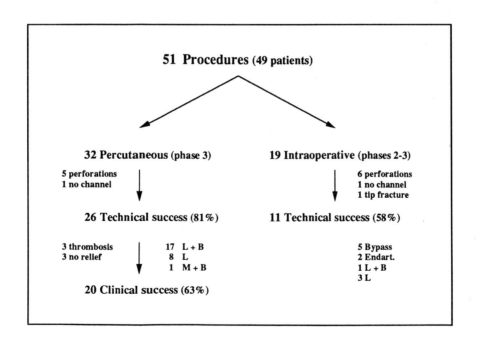

Fig. 7–4. Technical and clinical success of laser recanalization in 51 patients during phases 2 and 3. Endart., endarterectomy; L, laser angioplasty as sole therapy; L + B, laser recanalization followed by balloon angioplasty; M + B, mechanical recanalization (no activation of laser), followed by balloon angioplasty.

the ipsilateral common femoral artery [38]. Sequential guidewires and dilators were then used to place a 7–9 F internal diameter introducer sheath at the origin at the superficial femoral artery. Peripheral vein access was obtained and vital signs monitored noninvasively throughout the procedure. A bolus of heparin (5,000 U) was then given intrarterially followed by nitroglycerin (200 mcg) prior to the probe introduction.

A 2–2.5 mm sterile disposable hybrid probe was used to recanalize the arterial obstruction. The probe system and guidewire were backloaded into a 7 F thin-walled catheter [Cook, Bloomingdale, IN] with a hemostasis valve at the hub allowing for saline and/or contrast injection. The proximal end of the optical fiber was attached to a universal connector that was placed into the exit port of an argon-ion laser (HGM, Salt Lake City, UT, or Laser-Ionics, Orlando, FL).

The probe was tested prior to use by placing the tip in a nonreflective plastic bowl filled with saline solution and the beam delivered at 1 W for 1 s pulses at 0.2 s intervals. Goggles screening out the 488,514 nm wavelengths were used for eye protection. Under fluoroscopy, the catheter and probe units were then advanced together through the sheath to the level of the obstruction. The fiber tip was extruded about 2–3 cm from the tip of the catheter to avoid damage. Gentle pressure was applied to the probe to try to cross the obstruction mechanically. Such an event would be considered mechanical rather than as laser recanalization.

Activation of the laser was initiated at 5 W and 1-s pulses at 0.2-s intervals. If the obstruction was not penetrated, the power was progressively increased by 1–2 W increments per second to a maximum of 12 W. The probe was advanced with gentle pressure in a continuous fashion at a rate of approximately 1 cm/s. Probe sticking occurred rarely; however, in that event, the power output was increased and the probe was disengaged by pulling back during laser-pulse delivery. The probe was then reactivated and advanced in the same fashion as described above. Contrast injection was performed intermittently to test the progress of the recanalization process. Once the obstruction was crossed, a 0.016-in guidewire was advanced across the lesion and the probe and introducing catheter were pulled back while the probe was activated at a maximum of 12–14 W/s. At the end of the procedure, a repeat angiogram was performed. If the lumen diameter was < 50% of the "normal" vessel above and below the treated area, balloon angioplasty was performed to improve the channel diameter. If the lumen diameter was > 50%, then laser recanalization would be performed as a sole procedure.

Postrecanalization care. Patients received another bolus of heparin (5,000 U) after the sheath, and catheters were removed and hemostasis achieved. The patient was then maintained on heparin for a 24 h period in the recovery room and usually discharged within a 48-h period after the procedure.

Results. In phase 1, using a 2 mm hybrid probe, successful crossing of the obstructed segment was achieved in seven of the nine (78%) procedures attempted. Perforations occurred in two arteries (22%). On histology, no channels were seen in one artery and one graft, both occluded by fresh thrombus. The mean flow of the recanalized arterial segments, at mean pressure of 80 mm Hg, was 157 ± 102 cc/min through a lumen channel diameter of 3 ± 0.3 mm (measured on histologic cross sections). The debris collected during this procedure remained minimal (≤ 1 mg) [8].

During phases 2 and 3, a procedure was considered technically successful if the obstruction was crossed with angiographic improvement and without perforation. In phase 3, an immediate clinical success was defined as a procedure with improvement of symptoms and without complications (reclosure or urgent bypass surgery) in the first 24 h.

In phases 2 and 3, 49 patients were considered for treatment, and 51 procedures were performed (19 intraoperatively, 32 percutaneously) (see Fig. 7–4). It is important to emphasize that this group of patients all had total occlusions and had frequently associated conditions such as failed bypass grafts and excessive peripheral vascular disease.

Of the 19 procedures performed intraoperatively, 11 (58%) were technically successful and the recanalization procedure was completed by bypass surgery in five, endarterectomy in two, and balloon angioplasty in one. In this subgroup, only three patients had laser angioplasty as sole therapy. Perforations occurred in six patients (32%). In one patient, no adequate channel was achieved. Disengagement of the tip was seen once, and the patient was treated with bypass surgery.

In the 32 percutaneous procedures, technical success was achieved in 26 (81%) and clinical success in 20 (63%). Ankle-brachial index (ABI), recorded in 17 patients, improved from 0.57 ± 0.13 to 0.83 ± 0.15 (mean ± SD) (p<0.0001). Laser angioplasty was used as sole therapy in eight patients, and therapy was completed by balloon angioplasty in 17 others (Fig. 7–5). In one patient, the obstruction was crossed with mechanical pressure of the probe only (without laser activation) and the lumen was further improved with balloon angioplasty. Laser recanalization did not achieve angiographic improvement in one procedure and caused perforations in five (17%). None of the patients who

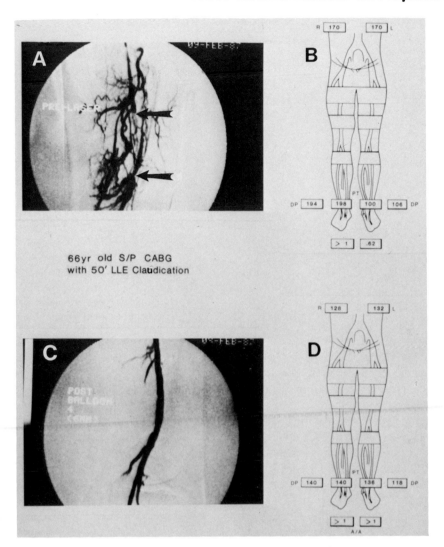

Fig. 7–5. **A,** Pre-laser angiogram of a totally occluded left superficial femoral artery (arrows). Collaterals are seen filling the distal vessel. This 66-year-old man had severe claudication at 50 ft. **B,** Pretreatment segmental pressures obtained by Doppler measurement. The left ankle-brachial index (ABI) is 0.62. **C,** Angiogram of the same artery as in A, after laser recanalization and balloon angioplasty. **D,** Posttreatment segmental pressures obtained by Doppler measurement. The left ABI is now > 1.

had arterial perforation developed hematoma at the perforated site that required urgent surgical repair or transfusions. Despite angiographic improvement after laser recanalization, three additional patients remained symptomatic and three patients reoccluded acutely.

Of the 12 patients with a failed attempt, five had subsequent bypass surgery, five were treated medically, and two patients, both attempted for limb salvage, were amputated. Amputation was considered a major complication in one patient who failed laser recanalization and underwent an attempt at balloon angioplasty the following day that was complicated by dissection and

thrombosis at the balloon-dilated site. The patient then underwent bypass surgery that resulted in thrombotic occlusion of the bypass graft 1 week later and transmetatarsal amputation was eventually required. Complications are reported in Table 7–2.

Clinical follow-up (mean 8.6 ± 4.0 months) is available in all the successful percutaneous procedures. Of 20 patients, 11 maintained symptom relief and nine had reappearance of their symptoms. Of these, seven were successfully treated either by balloon angioplasty (five) or bypass surgery (two) and two maintained on medical treatment.

TABLE 7–2. Complications in 51 Procedures (49 patients) in Phases 2–3

Complications	Intraoperative	Percutaneous
Major		
Amputation	0	1
Embolization	0	0
Thrombosis	0	3
Minor		
Perforations	6	5
Pain	0	10
Groin hematoma	0	6
Spasm (distal anterior tibia)	0	1
Other		
Probe disengagement	1	0

CONCLUSIONS

The current state-of-the-art using laser recanalization for the treatment of peripheral limb ischemia has been shown feasible, safe, and effective. Several limitations of this technique continue to require further refinement. These include the reduction of arterial perforation as well as the improvement in the luminal dimension. Also, thermal monitoring during recanalization using thermal systems with feedback control may be required in order to avoid thrombus formation seen with high levels of temperature ($> 300C°$) [39]. Spectral-monitoring to selectively ablate plaque may provide another approach to refine these techniques. With such improvements, it is not unreasonable to expect this technique to be used in stenosis of tortuous vessels such as the coronary arteries. The general consensus with the current systems, including the hybrid, laser probe, and Lastac, are that similar outcome and difficulties have been noted. All these systems currently require subsequent balloon angioplasty to enhance luminal dimensions. Only a few cases have been performed using the laser as the sole therapy with the hybrid system. Some of the patients followed over a long period of time still maintain symptom relief. It is important to bear in mind that these technologies are now part of an armamentarium that include stents, atherectomy, and mechanical recanalization devices. Which system will prove to be the ideal approach for a particular lesion such as atheromatous soft plaque, calcific plaque, or thrombus will require better understanding and further testing of these devices. Nevertheless, limited as current laser systems may be, they appear to be effective in converting a patient whose only option was bypass surgery to a less invasive alternative. From that perspective, these systems appear to serve a useful purpose.

REFERENCES

1. Abela GS, Normann S, Cohen D, Feldman RL, Geiser EA, Conti CR: Effects of Carbon dioxide, Nd-Yag, and argon laser radiation on coronary atheromatous plaques. Am J Cardiol 50:1199–1205, 1982.

2. Choy DSJ, Stertzer SH, Rotterdam HZ, Bruno MS: Laser coronary angioplasty: Experience with nine cadaver hearts. Am J Cardiol 50:1209–1211, 1982.

3. Lee G, Ikeda R, Herman I, Dwyer RM, Bass M, Hussein H, Kozina J, Mason DT: The qualitative effects of laser irradiation on human arteriosclerotic disease. Am Heart J 105:885–889, 1983.

4. Gerrity RG, Loop FD, Golding LAR, Ehrhart LA, Argenyi ZB: Arterial response to laser operation for removal of atherosclerotic plaques. J Thorac Cardiovasc Surg 85:409–421, 1983.

5. Abela GS, Crea F, Seeger JM, Franzini D, Fenech A, Normann SJ, Feldman RL, Pepine CJ, Conti CR: The healing process in normal canine arteries and in atherosclerotic monkey arteries after transluminal laser irradiation. Am J Cardiol 56:983–988, 1985.

6. Sanborn TA, Haudenschild CC, Garber GR, Ryan TJ, Faxon DP: Angiographic and histologic consequences of laser thermal angioplasty: comparison with balloon angioplasty. Circulation 75:1281–1286, 1987.

7. Isner JM, Donaldson RF, Deckelbaum LI, Clarke RH, Laliberte SM, Ucci AA, Salem DM, Konstam MA: The excimer laser: Gross, light microscopic and ultrastructural analysis of potential advantages for use in laser therapy of cardiovascular disease. J Am Coll Cardiol 6:1102–1109, 1985.

8. Abela GS, Seeger JM, Barbieri E, Franzini D, Fenech A, Pepine CJ, Conti CR: Laser angioplasty with angioscopic guidance in humans. J Am Coll Cardiol 8:184–192, 1986.

9. Abela GS, Crea F, Smith W, Pepine CJ, Conti CR: In vitro effects of argon laser radiation on blood: Quantitative and morphologic analysis. J Am Coll Cardiol 5:231–237, 1985.

10. Choy DSJ, Stertzer S, Loubeau JM, Kesseler H, Quilici P, Rotterdam H, Meltzer L: Embolization and vessel wall perforation in argon laser recanalization. Lasers Surg Med 5:297–308, 1985.

11. Sanborn TA, Faxon DP, Haudenschild CC, Ryan TJ: Experimental angioplasty: Circumferential distribution of laser thermal energy with a laser probe. J Am Coll Cardiol 5:934–938, 1985.

12. Abela GS, Normann SJ, Cohen DM, Franzini D, Feldman RL, Crea F, Fenech A, Pepine CJ, Conti CR: Laser recanalization of occluded atherosclerotic arteries in vivo and in vitro. Circulation 71:403–411, 1985.

13. Crea F, Abela GS, Fenech A, Smith W, Pepine CJ, Conti CR: Transluminal laser irradiation of coronary arteries in live dogs: An angiographic and morphologic study of acute effects. Am J Cardiol 57:171–174, 1986.

14. Crea F, Fenech A, Smith W, Conti CR, Abela GS: Laser recanalisation of acutely thrombosed coronary arteries in live dogs: Early results. J Am Coll Cardiol 6:1052–1056, 1985.

15. Nordstrom LA, Castaneda-Zuniga WR, Grewe DD, Schoster DVM: Laser enhanced transluminal angioplasty: The role of coaxial fiber placement. Semin Interven Radiol 3:47–52, 1986.

16. Seeger JM, Abela GS: Angioscopy as an adjunct to arterial reconstructive surgery: A preliminary report. J Vasc Surg 4:315–320, 1986.

17. Abela GS, Fenech A, Crea F, Conti CR: "Hot Tip": Another method of laser vascular recanalization. Lasers Surg Med 5:327–335, 1985.

18. Hussein H: A novel fiberoptic laser probe for treatment of occlusive vessel disease. Optical Laser Technol Med 605:59–66, 1986.

19. Van Gemert MJC, Verdaasdonk R, Stassen EG, Schets GACM, Gijsbers GHM, Bonnier JJ: Optical properties of human blood vessel wall and plaque. Lasers Surg Med 5:235–237, 1985.

20. Fenech A, Abela GS, Crea F, Smith W, Feldman RL, Conti CR: A comparative study of laser beam characteristics in blood and saline media. Am J Cardiol 55:1389–1392, 1985.

21. Litvack F, Grundfest W, Mohr F, Jakubowski A, Goldenberg T, Struhl B, Forrester JS: "Hot Tip" angioplasty by a novel radiofrequency catheter (abstract). Circulation 76:IV–47, 1987.

22. Lu DY, Leon MB, Bowman RL: A prototype catalytic thermal tip catheter: Design parameters and in vitro tissue studies (abstract). J Am Coll Cardiol 9:187A, 1987.

23. Fourrier JL, Brunetaud JM, Prat A, Marache P, Lablanche JM, Bretrand ME: Percutaneous laser angioplasty with sapphire tip. Lancet 1:105, 1987.

24. Grundfest W, Litvack F, Forrester JS, Goldenberg T, Swan HJC, Morgenstern L, Fishbein M, McDermid IS, Rider DM, Pacala TJ, Laudenslager JB: Laser ablation of human atherosclerotic plaque without adjacent tissue injury. J Am Coll Cardiol 5:929–933, 1985.

25. Abela GS, Barbieri E, Roxey T, Conti CR: Laser enhanced plaque atherolysis with tetracycline (abstract). Circulation 74:II–7, 1986.

26. Leon MB, Lu DY, Prevosti LG, Macy WW, Smith PD, Granovsky M, Bonner RF, Balaban RS: Human arterial surface fluorescence: Atherosclerotic plaque identification and effects of laser atheroma ablation. J Am Coll Cardiol 12:94–102, 1988.

27. Cothren RM, Hayes GB, Kramer JR, et al.: A multifiber catheter with an optical shield for laser angiosurgery. Lasers Life Sci 1:1, 1986.

28. Yock PG, Linker DT, Thapliyal HV, Arenson JW, Samstad S, Saether O, Angelsen BAJ: Real-time two-dimensional catheter ultrasound: A new technique for high-resolution intravascular imaging (abstract). J Am Coll Cardiol 11:130A, 1988.

29. Barbieri E, Abela GS, Khoury A, Roxey T, Conti CR: Coronary laser angioplasty in live dogs without perforation: Immediate and long term effects. Eur Heart J 8(2):154, 1987.

30. Abela GS, Barbieri E, Roxey T, Conti CR: Guided laser thermal angioplasty in coronary arteries of live dogs without perforation (abstract). Circulation 74:II–457, 1986.

31. Ginsburg R, Kim DS, Guthaner D, Toth J, Mitchell RS: Salvage of an ischemic limb by laser angioplasty: Description of a new technique. Clin Cardiol 7:54–58, 1984.

32. Geschwind H, Boussignac G, Teisseire B, Vieilledent C, Gaston A, Becquemin JP, Mayiolini P: Percutaneous transluminal laser angioplasty in man. Lancet 1:844, 1984.

33. Cumberland DC, Sanborn TA, Tayler DI, Moore DJ, Welsh CL, Greenfield AJ, Guben JK, Ryan TJ: Percutaneous laser thermal angioplasty: Initial clinical results with a laser probe in total peripheral artery occlusions. Lancet 1:1457, 1986.

34. Sanborn TA, Cumberland DC, Greenfield AJ, Welsh CL, Guben JK: Percutaneous laser thermal angioplasty: Initial results and one-year follow-up in 129 femoropopliteal lesions. Radiology 168:121–125, 1988.

35. Nordstrom LA, Castaneda-Zuniga WR, Young EG, Von Seggern KB: Direct argon laser exposure for recanalization of peripheral arteries: Early results. Radiology 168:359–364, 1988.

36. Hoffman RG, Abela GS, Friedl SE, Hojjatie B, Barbeau GR: Dosimetry of plaque ablation using thermal and thermal-optical probe systems (in press). Proceedings of SPIE-The International Society for Optical Engineering, Optical Fibers in Medicine IV, Volume 1067, 1989.

37. Barbieri E, Roxey T, Khoury A, Abela GS: Evaluation of optical properties and laser effects on arterial tissue using a microlens tipped optical fiber. Proceedings of SPIE- The International Society for Optical Engineering, Optical Fibers in Medicine II, Volume 713:166–169, 1986.

38. Abela GS, Seeger JM, Pry RS, Akins EW, Siragusa RJ, Barbieri E, Jablonski S: Percutaneous laser recanalization of totally occluded human peripheral arteries: A technical approach. Dynamic Cardiovasc Imag 1:302–308, 1988.

39. Barbieri E, Abela GS, Khoury A, Conti CR: Temperature characteristics of laser thermal probes in the coronary circulations of dogs (abstract). Circulation 76:IV–409, 1987.

8. Techniques and Experience in Laser Angioplasty at the Texas Heart Institute

D. Richard Leachman, M.D.

INTRODUCTION

In recent years, there has been an intense interest in the use of laser energy to treat patients with vascular disease, both in peripheral vascular beds and in coronary arteries. This interest has come about because of recognized deficiencies with the balloon angioplasty technique, including the difficulty in recanalizing total occlusions, treating patients with diffuse disease, and the unacceptably high rate of restenosis. Current laser angioplasty techniques allow reliable recanalization of total occlusions in peripheral arteries and may have an impact on restenosis through debulking the lesion or through a thermal effect. As the technology continues to evolve, the applications and clinical utility will likewise expand.

Patients referred for laser angioplasty of peripheral arterial occlusions are generally elderly (mean age in our series is 65 years) and often have occlusive disease of other vascular beds. Many also have associated medical problems such as diabetes, renal insufficiency, or congestive heart failure. Diagnostic angiography of multiple vascular beds is required for complete evaluation of these patients even though they often do not tolerate angiographic procedures well. For those patients with diabetes or renal insufficiency, the usual attention given to volume status and adequate hydration is even more important.

DIAGNOSTIC ANGIOGRAPHY FOR PATIENT SELECTION

The decision to proceed with laser angioplasty depends on the presence of symptoms and anatomical status as defined by diagnostic angiography. Routine runoff studies are usually adequate for determining the location and severity of vascular occlusions; however, other relevant anatomic details may become apparent by use of selective angiography. For example, selective angiograms may allow more adequate determination of a vascular occlusion through better filling. In addition, selective angiography allows more detailed definition of the entrance into an occlusion, which is of critical importance in laser procedures. The entrance may be symmetrical and central, or it may be eccentric. Furthermore, occlusions frequently begin just distal to a collateral vessel. Angled angiographic views can help to define this crucial anatomic point.

Most angiography of the peripheral arteries is performed from the femoral approach, which produces very adequate studies. I prefer the brachial approach because with this approach good-quality selective angiograms of the femoral arteries can be obtained, and it allows easy angiographic access to other vasculature, such as coronary and carotid areas. With the brachial approach, diagnostic angiography can be accomplished without trauma to either femoral artery. This is advantageous in cases wherein the femoral arteries will later be used for access during laser procedures. Occasionally, I will proceed with routine balloon angioplasty of iliac stenoses from a brachial approach during the diagnostic study. The brachial approach helps to prepare patients with superficial femoral artery occlusion for a laser procedure by superficial femoral artery antegrade puncture the following day.

RESULTS

We have performed laser-assisted balloon angioplasty in 167 lesions in 130 patients; the overall success rate is 83%. The success rates vary, depending on the percentage of stenosis and the length of the occlusion. The success rate for stenosis is 98% (49 of 50). The success rate for total occlusions less than 10 cm in length is 80%, and for those longer than 10 cm, 50%. Success rates do not appear to be affected by the type of vessel occluded (Table 8–1). The successful outcomes with use of laser-assisted balloon angioplasty are similar for iliac, superficial femoral, popliteal, and trifurcation vessels. We have also completed the laser procedure from the brachial approach in 11 patients, with a success rate

Laser Angioplasty, pages 59–76
© 1989 Alan R. Liss, Inc.

TABLE 8–1. Success Rates According to Type of Vessel Occluded

Arterial segments	No.	Success rate (%)
Iliac	17	85
Superficial femoral	129	78
Popliteal	10	90
Tibial	8	100
Common femoral	3	33

TABLE 8–2. Complications

Type	Probe-related	Procedure-related
Thrombus	0	0
Embolism	0	2
Dissection	0	1
Perforation	20	0
Hematoma	1	2
Emergency surgery	0	3
Death	0	1
Early reocclusion	0	8

of 83%. This is not significantly different from the success rate using the femoral approach (82%). Good immediate angiographic and clinical results were shown in 11 patients who underwent laser-assisted balloon angioplasty to avoid limb amputation (limb-salvage patients). The immediate success rate in these patients was a surprising 91%, and at 6 month follow-up, the limb salvage in this group remained at 81% (9 of 11 patients). In this patient group, the preprocedure ankle-brachial index was 0.37; after the procedure, it was 0.73.

COMPLICATIONS

Perforations

The incidence of complications in our patients has been acceptable (Table 8–2). There have been 20 perforations in 167 attempts (12%), most of which occurred in the first 50 cases. According to serial hematocrit levels and hemodynamic follow-up, none of the perforations resulted in significant blood loss. The area of perforation was explored in several patients who had elective surgery after the failed laser angioplasty. The typical observation has been the presence of a small perivascular hematoma, and the site of perforation in the artery has not been discernible. The benign nature of perforations in peripheral arteries may be attributed to a relatively small probe (2 mm diameter) causing a hole in a segment of artery under generally low perfusion pressure. The thermal nature of the laser probe

may tend to seal the hole in the artery. Whether the benign nature of these perforations will hold true in intraabdominal or intracoronary vessels is doubtful, particularly if larger probes are used. No perforations have occurred when the probe has been used over a guidewire.

Groin Hematomas and Embolization

Two patients developed large groin hematomas following antegrade puncture of the femoral artery; one (0.6%) of those required surgery for hemostasis. Two other patients (1.2%) had emboli to the trifurcation following balloon angioplasty of superficial femoral artery lesions. Both patients had total occlusions that were successfully recanalized with the laser probe, but embolized only after subsequent balloon angioplasty. Both patients did well after Fogarty embolectomy. Histologic examination of the retrieved material revealed semiorganized thrombus that was neither acute (and potentially treatable with thrombolytic agents) nor chronic.

POSTANGIOPLASTY HISTOLOGY

One patient died 8 h after an angioplasty procedure. The patient had a short (4 cm) subtotal occlusion of the superficial femoral artery. It was easily recanalized with a 2 mm laser probe and subsequently dilated with a 5 mm balloon. The angiographic result was good (Fig. 8–1). The patient also had a more proximal stenosis in the superficial femoral artery, which was dilated with a 5 mm balloon without prior laser therapy. The angiographic lesions and results, which are shown in Figure 8–2, were considered quite adequate even though the angiographic appearance of an intimal split is obvious. Histologic examination of these two arterial segments demonstrates the typical features of postballoon angioplasty trauma with intimal tears and significant compromise of the arterial lumen (Fig. 8–3), contrary to the angiographic appearance. In contrast, the segment treated with a 2 mm laser probe prior to balloon inflation shows a remarkable absence of intimal trauma and impressive symmetric enlargement of the arterial lumen (Fig. 8–4). The histologic evidence of thermal effect is limited to the intima. Although this histologic-angiographic correlation is represented in only one case, the histologic difference is impressive and tends to support the theory that the "debulking" (removing a portion of the occlusive atheroma) or thermal effect may lead to better early results, which may conceivably lead to better long-term results.

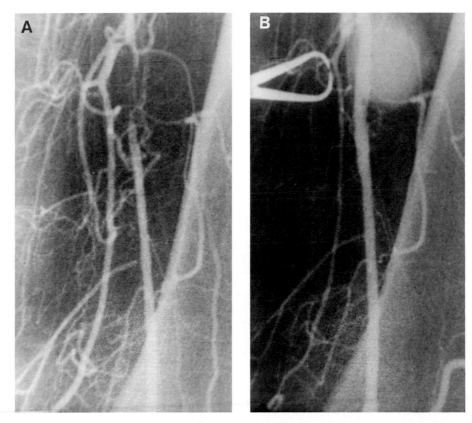

Fig. 8–1. **A,** A short subtotal occlusion of the superficial femoral artery. **B,** Good angiographic result following laser recanalization with a 2 mm laser probe and subsequent angioplasty with a 5 mm balloon.

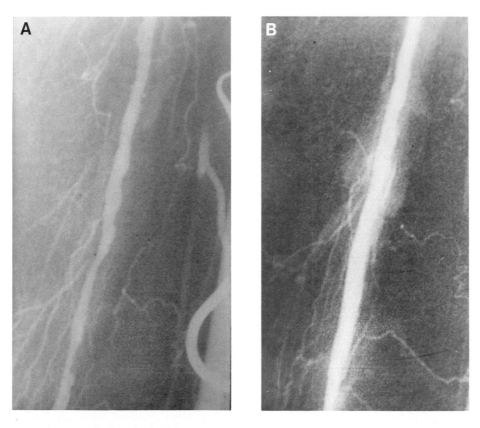

Fig. 8–2. **A,** Stenosis of the superficial femoral artery. **B,** Good angiographic result after angioplasty with a 5 mm balloon (no laser recanalization).

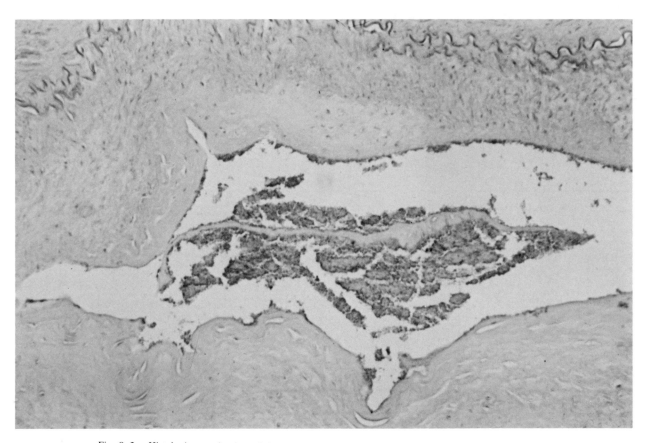

Fig. 8–3.   Histologic examination of the arterial stenosis treated only by balloon angioplasty demonstrates significant intimal tearing and compromise of the lumen.

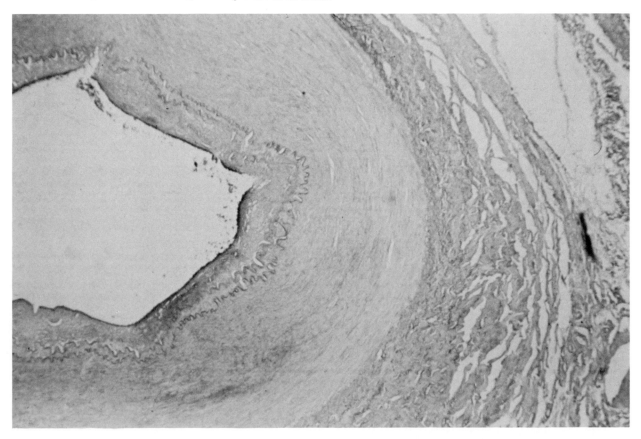

Fig. 8–4.   Histologic examination of the subtotal occlusion in which a 2 mm laser probe was used for recanalization, followed by balloon angioplasty. Minimal intimal tearing and only superficial thermal effect is shown.

CONSIDERATIONS OF ARTERIAL ANATOMY

In my experience with laser-assisted balloon angioplasty, I have identified some specific problems related to arterial anatomy, which may be important in the practice of this technique. The ideal total occlusion is short, with a symmetrical, concentric entrance in a noncalcified straight arterial segment. This type of case, however, is as difficult to find as the ideal "Gruntzig" coronary angioplasty case.

Ideal Case

The example shown in Figure 8–5 illustrates an almost ideal model of total occlusion. It is a 4 cm total occlusion located in a fairly straight segment of the superficial femoral artery. There is no calcium visible in the occlusion under fluoroscopic examination. The entrance into the occlusion is almost perfectly symmetrical, and it begins about 1 cm distal to a major collateral branch. In this type of case, after an 8 F sheath is placed antegrade over a guidewire into the superficial femoral artery, 5,000–10,000 U of heparin are administered, according to the size of the patient and its effect on the activated clotting time, which is monitored in the catheterization lab. In this particular case, a 2.0 "plus" laser probe was advanced through the occlusion by using 10 W of argon laser power. The lumen was partially recanalized, as illustrated in Figure 8–5B, and a 5 mm balloon could be passed easily into the lesion over a guidewire as seen in Figure 8–5C. The artery was then dilated, and the final angiographic result was excellent (Fig. 8–5D). In this case, as is usual following laser angioplasty, there was minimal angiographic evidence of intimal tearing or disruption.

After a typical procedure, the sheaths are pulled within 1–4 h, depending on the postprocedure-activated clotting time and the size of the femoral artery. If the artery is small and there is concern that the sheath may significantly impair flow through the artery, then the tendency is to pull the sheath earlier to avoid thrombotic problems in the superficial femoral artery. Generally, the patient is given heparin for 24 h after the procedure and is discharged on aspirin and persantine.

The Brachial Approach

The most common percutaneous approaches for laser angioplasty of peripheral occlusions have been antegrade entry into the common femoral artery for superficial femoral artery, popliteal, or trifurcation disease

and retrograde entry into the common femoral artery for iliac occlusions. In the majority of cases, these approaches work very well. In some circumstances, however, an alternative approach is desirable. For example, when the occlusion for laser angioplasty involves the common femoral or the proximal portion of the superficial femoral artery, percutaneous placement of a sheath is usually not possible.

If the occlusion is in the iliac artery, the theoretical alternative is to approach it either from the contralateral groin or from a brachial approach. The contralateral femoral approach might be difficult because of concern about sufficient support for advancing the laser probe and balloon. To reach an occlusion from this approach, the acute angle at the aortic bifurcation must be passed with a guiding catheter. Although this can usually be accomplished without great difficulty, there is an important loss in "pushability" once an acute angle has been traversed with any catheter. Since the ability to recanalize total occlusions depends on both thermal and mechanical properties of the laser probe, it would probably be difficult to generate enough forward force on the probe to recanalize occlusions from this approach.

In contrast, recanalizing the iliac, common femoral, and proximal superficial femoral artery occlusions from the brachial approach has been successful. Generally, a guiding catheter can be advanced easily to the origin of the occlusion and then the laser probe can be advanced, just as a percutaneous transluminal coronary angioplasty (PTCA) catheter is advanced. The guiding catheter usually allows sufficient support to pass the laser probe through the lesion. An 8 F large-lumen guiding catheter will allow easy passage of the 1.5 mm or the 1.7 mm laser probes. The current preference in these cases is the 1.7 mm "sidehold" probe, which has a central lumen for contrast injections or guidewire placement.

This approach is illustrated in Figure 8–6 in which there was a short occlusion of the common femoral artery that could not be crossed with a guidewire (Fig. 8–6A). A brachial guiding catheter (8.3 F) was advanced near the origin of the occlusion of the common femoral artery, and a 1.5 mm laser probe was advanced through the occlusion (Fig. 8–6B), creating a small channel (Fig. 8–6C). This allowed passage of a .014 in. coronary guidewire and subsequent balloon catheter to adequately dilate the artery (Fig. 8–6D).

Another situation wherein the brachial approach is useful is in patients in whom multiple dilatations are necessary. In the case illustrated in Figure 8–7, balloon dilatation of both renal arteries was performed at the time of laser recanalization of an occluded right femoral artery. The brachial approach provided the best guiding approach to accomplish all these procedures at the same time. In this case, a brachial guiding catheter with a

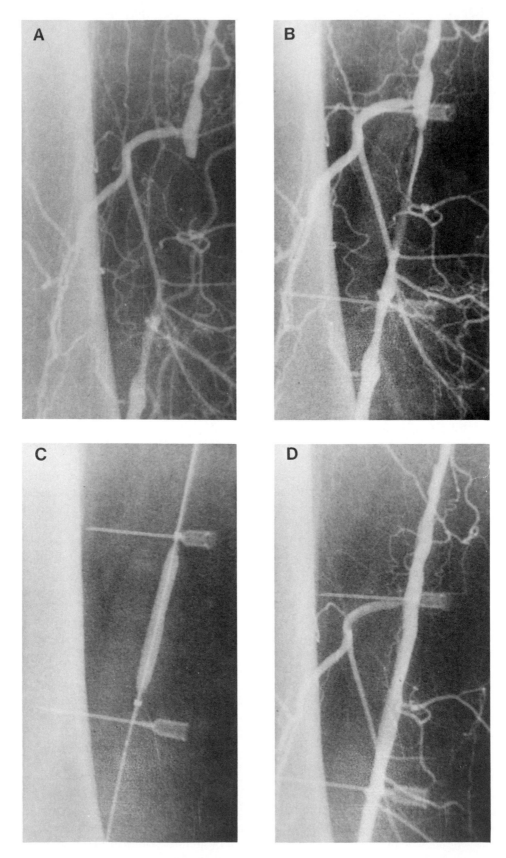

Fig. 8–5.   **A,** A 4 cm total occlusion of the superficial femoral artery. **B,** Recanalized channel through the occlusion following passage of a 2.0 plus laser probe. **C,** A 5 mm balloon inflated in the lesion. **D,** Final angiographic result showing minimal evidence of intimal tearing.

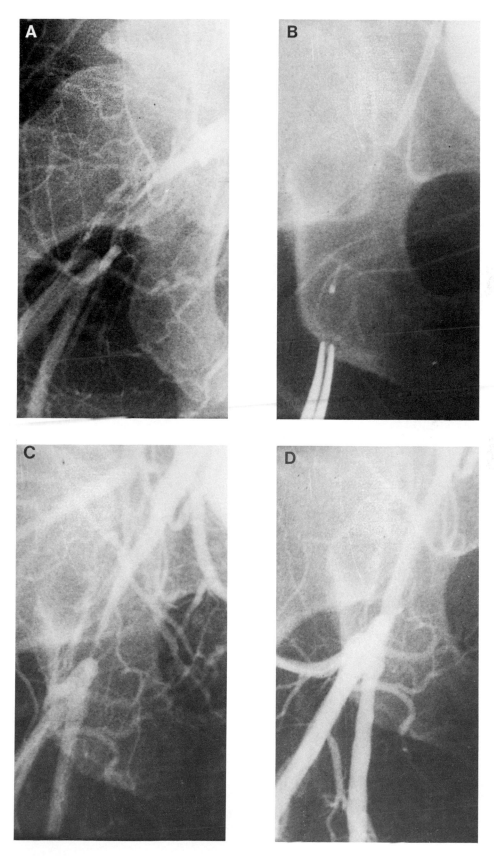

Fig. 8–6. **A,** A short total occlusion of the common femoral artery. **B,** A Stertzer guiding catheter tip providing support in the common femoral artery, after a 1.5 mm laser probe has crossed the occlusion. **C,** A very small recanalized channel through the occlusion demonstrating adequate passage of a balloon over a wire. **D,** Final angiographic result after balloon dilatation.

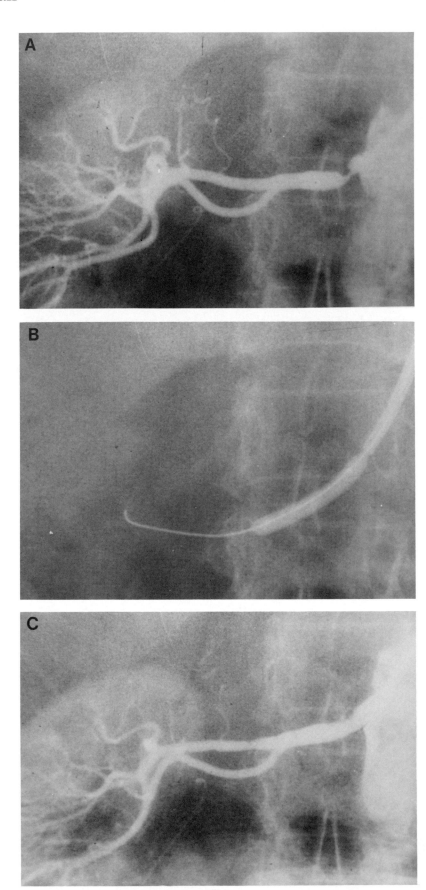

Fig. 8–7, **A–C.** **A,** Right renal artery stenosis. **B,** A balloon catheter inflated in the stenosis with brachial guiding catheter support. **C,** Final angiographic result after balloon angioplasty of the right renal artery stenosis.

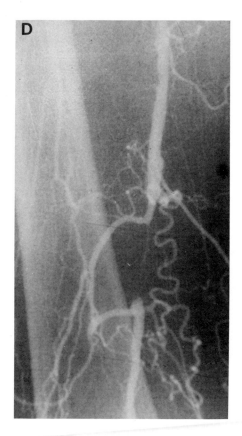 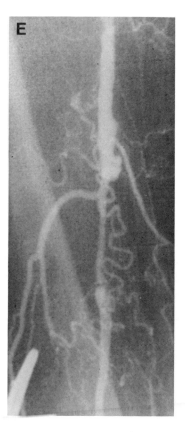 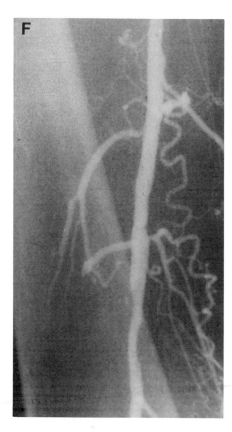

Fig. 8–7, **D–F.** **D,** A short occlusion of the mid-right superficial femoral artery. **E,** The recanalized channel through the occlusion after passage with a 1.5 mm laser probe. **F,** Final angiographic result after balloon dilatation.

coronary balloon system was used to dilate the renal artery stenoses (Fig. 8–7 A–C). Then, in order to recanalize the superficial femoral artery occlusion, the brachial guiding catheter (8.3 F) was advanced to the superficial femoral artery near the occlusion. Recanalization was then achieved with a 1.5 mm laser probe and was followed by balloon dilatation for a good angiographic result (Fig. 8–7 D–F).

SPECIFIC ANATOMIC PROBLEMS

Long Occlusions

A major problem in case selection is presented by the patient with the long superficial femoral artery occlusion. As shown in earlier statistics, success rates with laser-assisted balloon angioplasty are inversely related to lesion length. There has been a significant decline in success rates for cases involving lesions longer than 10 cm. This, in part, relates to the difficulty in "steering" a probe through a long total occlusion without becoming subintimal. It is also probably true that longer total

occlusions tend to be older than are shorter ones. The longer occlusions may be more fibrotic or calcified and thus more difficult to vaporize with the laser probe. A case of successful laser recanalization of a long total occlusion is illustrated in Figure 8–8. This occlusion measured 14 cm in length, and we had an excellent angiographic result. The patient also has had a good long-term result ($> 1\frac{1}{2}$ yr), probably due in part to excellent distal runoff.

Calcified Lesions

It is not uncommon to identify, under fluoroscopy, calcium in occlusions selected for laser treatment. A small amount of calcium in an occlusion or stenosis does not usually preclude the possibility of recanalization with the laser probe; however, significant amounts of calcium in a lesion can cause difficulty. Of the 167 lesions attempted, a large number were calcified, but only two of these occlusions could not be crossed with

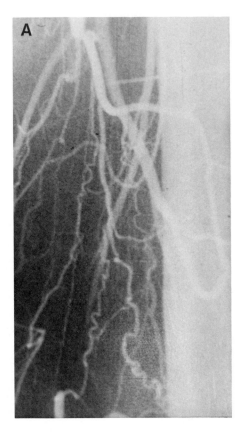

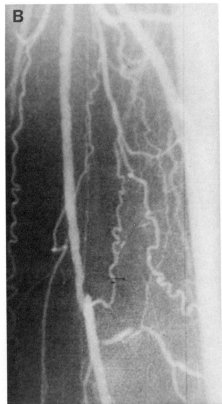

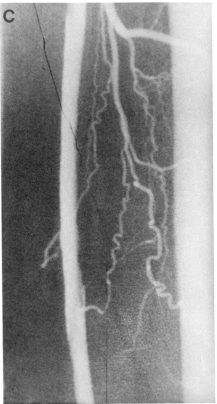

Fig. 8–8. **A,** A long (14 cm) total occlusion of the superficial femoral artery. **B,** The recanalized channel through the occlusion after passage with a 2.0 plus laser probe. **C,** Excellent final angiographic result after balloon dilatation.

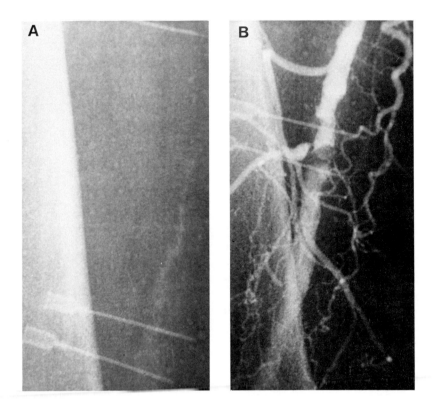

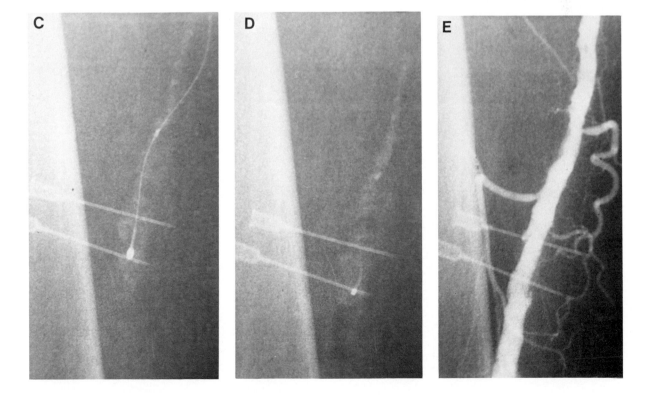

Fig. 8–9.   **A,** Heavy calcium deposits in the superficial femoral artery between the needles. **B,** Angiographic demonstration of a short total occlusion of the superficial femoral artery. **C,** Occlusion after failure of penetration with a 2.0 plus laser probe at maximum power with significant force as seen by the flexion of the .035 in. plus wire. **D,** Occlusion after failure of recanalization with 1.5 mm laser probe. **E,** Final angiographic result after balloon dilatation.

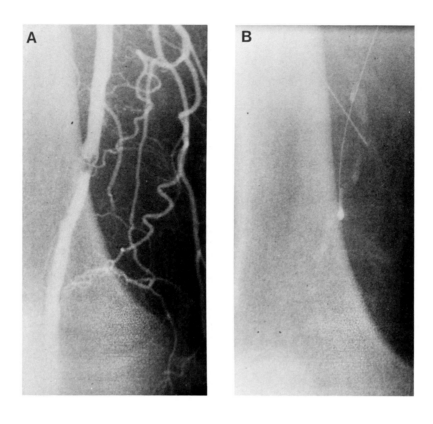

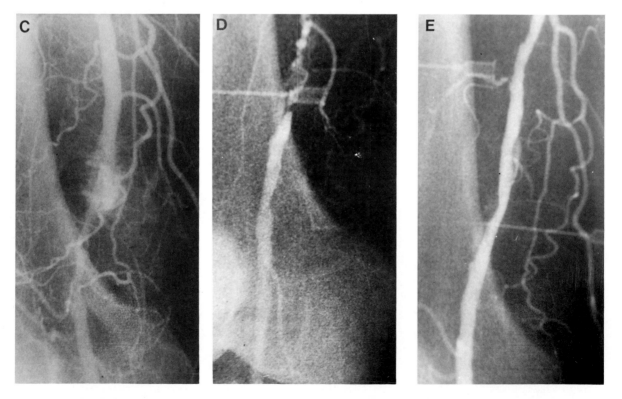

Fig. 8–10.   **A,** A very asymmetric stenosis of the superficial femoral artery. **B,** A 2.0 plus laser probe deviating medially and perforating the artery. **C,** Angiographic demonstration of vessel perforation. **D,** Angiographic appearance of the same artery 3 months later. **E,** Final angiographic result after balloon dilatation.

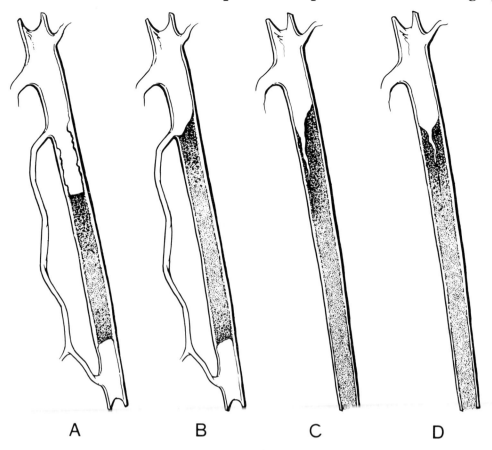

Fig. 8–11.   **A,** Occlusion beginning distal to the origin of a collateral.
B, Occlusion beginning at the origin of a collateral branch. **C,** Occlusion
with an eccentric entrance. **D,** Occlusion with a concentric entrance.

the laser probe. One was a very short, heavily calcified total occlusion of the superficial femoral artery (Fig. 8–9). In our initial attempt to recanalize the occlusion, we used a 2.0 plus probe with a .035 in. stiff wire fixed alongside the fiberoptic catheter. This probe was stiff enough to be pushed with a significant amount of force. Even with maximum recommended laser power, however, this probe could not be passed through the occlusion. Subsequent attempts with use of a 1.5 mm laser probe at maximum recommended power also failed. The lesion was ultimately passed with the stiff end of an .014 in. coronary guidewire followed by a 3 mm balloon. This created a lumen large enough to cross with a larger 6 mm balloon for an adequate final result. New technology that is currently under development may allow these lesions to be recanalized with the laser. Lower-profile steerable laser wires may allow some of these calcified or "hard" lesions to be more easily passed.

Asymmetric Lesions

Lesion symmetry is another important variable when considering laser recanalization of a subtotal or total occlusion.

The symmetry of a totally occluded arterial segment is more difficult to appreciate angiographically than that of a subtotal occlusion. In extremely asymmetric lesions, particularly if they are calcified or very hard, the laser probe may deflect off the hard atheromatous plaque and perforate the opposite arterial wall as illustrated in Figure 8–10. This case represents the only one we had of subtotal occlusion in which laser recanalization failed. The lesion was extremely asymmetric and calcified. During attempts to pass a 2 mm laser probe, the tip was deflected and perforated the opposite wall. This patient was treated before guidewires were available for use with laser probes. If such a case were to be done today, first a guidewire, and then the probe, would be passed across the stenosis. With this "over-the-wire" technique, there have been no perforations in peripheral vessels or in coronary arteries. Fortunately, the patient returned 3 months after the initial laser attempt, and a longer stenosis was successfully treated.

Total occlusions are obviously more difficult to assess with regard to symmetry. The underlying stenosis that precedes the total occlusion can be symmetrical or asymmetrical; unless a portion of the occlusion is densely calcified, however, the symmetry of lesions in total occlusions is virtually impossible to assess.

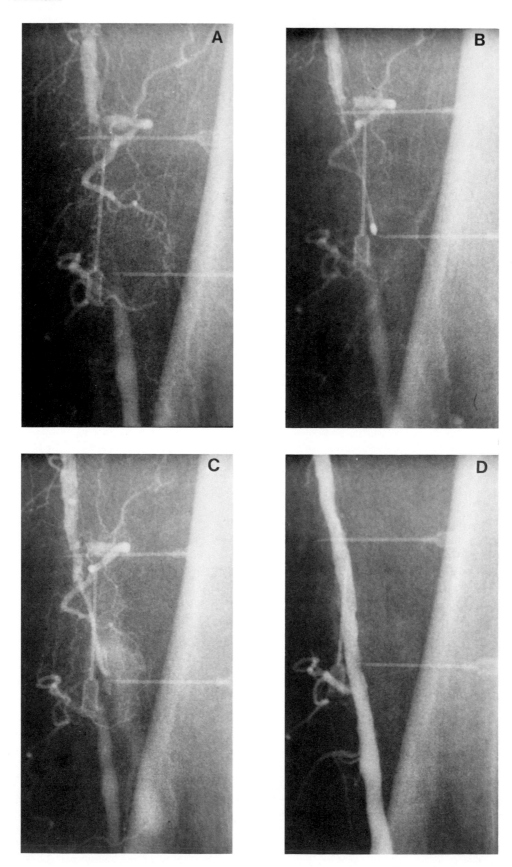

Fig. 8–12.   **A,** A 4 cm total occlusion of the superficial femoral artery with an eccentric entry into the occlusion. It is lateral (toward the femur). **B,** Perforation of the artery through the lateral wall with a 2.0 plus probe.   **C,** Angiographic demonstration of the perforation. **D,** Final angiographic result once the true lumen has been reentered with the balloon. The perforation is sealed.

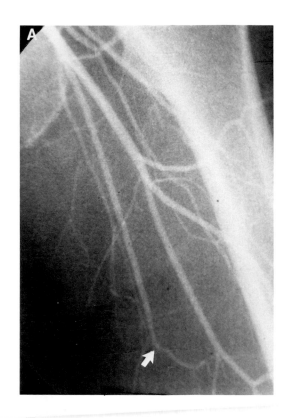

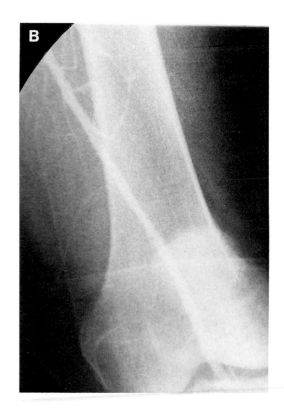

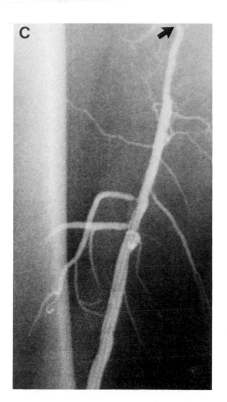

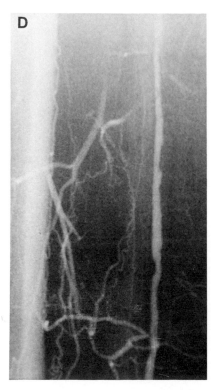

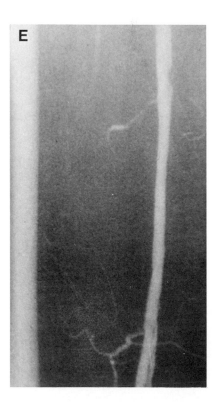

Fig. 8–13. **A,** A very small diffusely diseased superficial femoral artery with an ostial stenosis and a mid superficial femoral artery occlusion. The superficial femoral artery terminates flush into a collateral (arrow). **B,** View of a popliteal artery that is larger and less diseased than the proximal superficial femoral artery. **C,** Angiogram demonstrating the distal termination of the superficial femoral occlusion. With the patient in the prone position, a sheath is placed in the popliteal artery. The distal end of the occlusion is seen on the top of the figure (arrow). **D,** Angiographic demonstration of the recanalized channel through the superficial femoral artery occlusion by retrograde passage of the laser probe. **E,** Final angiographic result after balloon angioplasty.

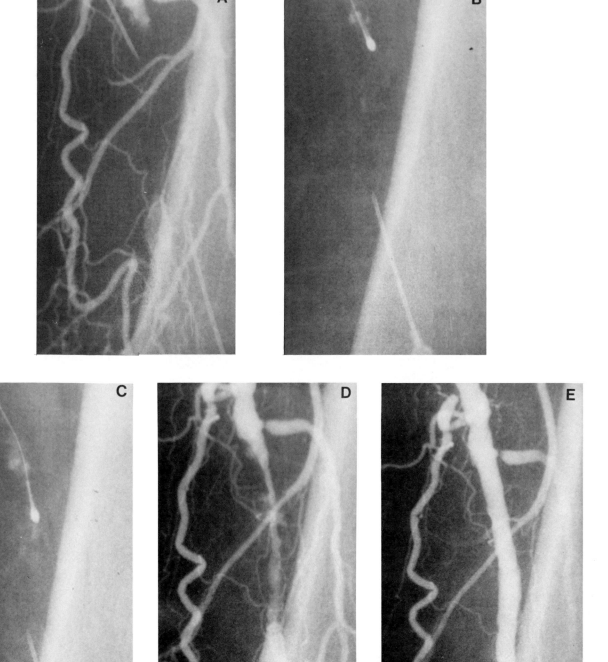

Fig. 8–14. **A,** A 6 cm total occlusion involving Hunter's canal. **B,** A 2.0 plus probe that is advanced without shaping the wire. It appears to be somewhat laterally deviated. **C,** The probe tip redirected toward the true lumen by shaping the plus wire with a gentle S curve. **D,** The recanalized channel following passage of the 2.0 plus laser probe. **E,** Final angiographic result after balloon angioplasty.

Entry into the Occlusion

The success or failure of laser recanalization may depend in part on how the laser probe enters the occlusion. Therefore, one of the angiographic details that requires close attention when selecting patients for laser angioplasty is the angle for entry into the total occlusion. To determine this, angled views are frequently taken during diagnostic angiography. The beginning of an occlusion may be flush without an entry channel, it may originate flush with a collateral branch, or the entry channel may be either symmetric or eccentric in the artery (Fig. 8–11). If the laser probe enters the occlusion in an eccentric fashion, the likelihood is greater that the probe will eventually pass subintimally or perforate as it is advanced. If the probe enters the occlusion centrally, then subintimal passage of the laser probe is less likely unless significant asymmetry or vessel tortuosity is present.

The importance of the entrance into the lesion is illustrated in Figure 8–12. This patient had a short (5 cm) total occlusion of the superficial femoral artery, which initially appeared to be an excellent case for laser recanalization. The entrance into the occlusion, however, was eccentric in the artery and in the illustration can be seen deviating laterally (toward the bone). The laser probe followed that channel and eventually perforated the artery. It was possible in this case to steer back into the true lumen and ultimately seal the perforation. My approach to the issue of how the laser probe enters the artery has been to slowly advance a 2.0 plus laser probe into the vessel for a few centimeters and then reassess its position by using contrast injections. If it appears to be notably deviating off center, it is removed from the artery. Then, the .035 plus wire is shaped with a gentle curve to allow steerability as it is advanced through the occlusion. Once the laser probe has clearly passed subintimally or has perforated, it is not impossible to reenter the true lumen (as shown in Fig. 8–12), but it is very difficult.

The Popliteal Approach

It is not uncommon for total occlusions, particularly in the superficial femoral artery, to originate at the point of takeoff of a collateral branch, as illustrated in Figure 8–11B. These occlusions may be difficult to recanalize with the laser probe because the probe may tend to enter the collateral channel rather than the occlusion itself. Laser energy applied at that point may perforate the collateral vessel. When an occlusion originates at a collateral, multiple angled views of the occlusion are obtained angiographically to pinpoint where the collateral

begins and where the occlusion begins. Some collaterals branch off at 90° angles and, consequently, are more difficult to define angiographically. Collaterals may also superimpose with the occlusion in some views. This is why angled views are important. Even when angled views adequately separate the collateral from the occluded artery, however, it still may be impossible to prevent the laser probe from entering the collateral.

In cases such as these, it is sometimes advisable to approach these occlusions from below, via the popliteal artery, as shown in Figure 8–13. In this case, a diagnostic angiogram revealed a 10 cm occlusion of the superficial femoral artery that originated at a collateral. The superficial femoral artery terminated flush into the collateral at an angle that would have been difficult to avoid entering with the laser probe (Fig. 8–13A). The proximal superficial femoral artery was very small, and the popliteal artery was larger and less diseased (Fig. 8–13B). This occlusion was approached from the popliteal artery. Via the percutaneous method, a sheath was placed retrograde into the popliteal artery (Fig. 8–13C) and the laser probe was advanced retrograde through the occlusion (Fig. 8–13D), avoiding the collateral altogether after balloon dilation (Fig. 13E), with an adequate angiographic result. This approach is somewhat cumbersome, particularly since proximal contrast injections are not possible, and it is reserved for situations in which an antegrade approach has clear disadvantages.

Tortuosity in Hunter's Canal

Another anatomic situation resulting in difficult laser recanalization is that of an occlusion involving Hunter's canal. This segment of the superficial femoral artery is mildly tortuous and is associated with a higher incidence of procedural failures due to perforation or subintimal passing of the probe. The football-shaped tip of the laser probe probably contributes to the fact that this device tends to stay in the true lumen as it passes total occlusions. However, tortuous arterial segments may result in a greater tendency for the laser probe to become eccentric in the vessel wall or to perforate. One way to prevent this is to shape the .035 in. plus wire of the 2.0 plus probe and then torque it to steer through these tortuous segments. When the wire is shaped, a gentle C curve or S curve is fixed to it, because as pressure is applied to the probe, these curves become further exaggerated, depending on the amount of pressure applied. As illustrated in Figure 8–14, the S curve may help keep the probe intraluminal in occlusions involving tortuous arteries, such as in the Hunter's canal area. This is another situation wherein a highly steerable and shapeable laser wire could be very useful.

CONCLUSIONS

Our experience with laser recanalization of arterial occlusions in peripheral arteries has been successful, with a low complication rate. When performed percutaneously, it offers the patient the same advantages over surgery as balloon angioplasty: primarily, a shorter hospital stay and a shorter recuperation time. This technology will certainly evolve quickly in the next few years, and we are likely to witness an improvement in already acceptable success rates, as well as broader indications for performing this procedure.

9. Surgical Laser Recanalization Techniques

Edward B. Diethrich, M.D.

INTRODUCTION

The successful clinical use of laser thermal energy to vaporize occlusive atherosclerotic lesions in the peripheral and coronary circulations has garnered international attention. Pioneered a few years ago by cardiologists and interventional radiologists [1–14], the use of lasers from a variety of sources appeared promising in the recanalization of obstructed arteries. However, the surgeon's role until now has been confined to "standby" status, awaiting either an unsuccessful outcome or a failed procedure complicated by an untoward event requiring immediate operation.

This territoriality was certainly understandable in view of the historical development of angioplasty. It was the nonsurgical specialists who created and refined the techniques for angiographic visualization of every vascular distribution. Their ingenuity was responsible for applying a balloon to the tip of the catheter, giving birth to percutaneous peripheral and coronary balloon angioplasty. The resulting explosion of practitioners of this technique left little doubt that improvements were not far off. The addition of a laser beam to the catheter was a natural development in the evolution of this exciting therapeutic process. However, these nonsurgical specialists faced an access limitation imposed by their percutaneous pathway, restricting their application of laser angioplasty to uncomplicated arterial occlusions and short, high-grade stenoses.

The surgeon's reluctance to pursue percutaneous angioplastic techniques was a product of his/her training. Under most circumstances, surgeons had not found it advantageous to become familiar with therapeutic modalities in which catheters and angiographic control were required.

In the early 1970s, the usefulness of intraoperative angiographic control in both peripheral and coronary procedures was introduced at the Arizona Heart Institute [15–17]. An operating room was equipped with a C-arm radiographic unit and Kifa table to permit intraoperative visualization before and after recanalization procedures. This vast experience in intraoperative angiography facilitated the introduction of laser technology at our institution, either as a sole modality or in conjunction with other vascular operative procedures [18–23].

Since the February 1987 FDA approval of laser-assisted angioplasty, our facility has offered this technique to all patients with symptomatic peripheral occlusive disease. Our initial selection of laser-assisted vascular recanalization is predicated on three assumptions.

First, laser energy should penetrate even a totally occluded arterial segment, establishing at least a central channel through which a dilating balloon catheter could be introduced to fully expand the artery.

Second, the vascular surgeon has unrestricted capabilities to gain entry to any artery, even in the presence of extensive occlusive disease. This circumvents the access limitation of the nonsurgical specialists.

Third, in most cases, a failed laser angioplasty procedure can be converted to a classical revascularization operation, culminating in a successful outcome for the patient.

As both an introduction to surgeons seeking familiarization with the technology and as evidence for the laser's eminent applicability to the field of vascular surgery, we offer the protocols, equipment, techniques, and patient-care requirements we have devised and employed during our experience in over 700 laser-assisted peripheral vascular recanalizations. The growing applications for laser ablation of atherosclerotic plaque have become more and more successful, and their intraoperative use will certainly offer an entirely new armamentarium for the vascular surgeon. Undoubtedly, the information presented today will soon change, as the research efforts in this dynamic field bring forth still more advantageous refinements in technique and instrumentation.

PATIENT SELECTION AND PREOPERATIVE EVALUATION

All patients seen in our clinic with symptoms of lower limb arterial insufficiency (hip, thigh, or calf claudication; rest pain; ulceration; or threatened limb loss) are

Laser Angioplasty, pages 77–91

considered candidates for laser angioplasty. This is possible because the procedure will be performed in an operating room by vascular surgeons who have the capability to revascularize the limb using conventional surgical techniques should the laser fail to penetrate the lesion(s) and create, either solely or in combination with a balloon catheter, a satisfactory vascular channel.

An arterial Doppler examination (preferably with exercise if symptoms and physical examination permit) is made to establish a baseline ankle/brachial systolic pressure index (ABI) for use in evaluating long-term patency. Documentation of the lower extremity arterial system is accomplished using translumbar, retrograde, or antegrade arteriography, depending on the location of the lesions: translumbar aortography and antegrade studies are used if both iliac arteries are totally occluded or both common femoral arteries (CFAs) are severely diseased.

Although the treatment plan in these patients is to use laser-assisted angioplasty rather than conventional surgical procedures, all patients electing laser angioplasty are informed that a bypass procedure or endarterectomy may be performed when necessary and possible if the laser technique fails to establish an open vessel. Patients electing laser angioplasty are started on 325 mg/day of aspirin and 75 mg dipyridamole t.i.d. 48 h before surgery.

Of course, certain categories of patients are scheduled for combined laser and surgical revascularization from the onset due to the nature of their lesions. For example, in the case of CFA and profunda femoris lesions with disease in the superficial femoral artery (SFA), the procedures used would be CFA and profunda endarterectomies, profundaplasty, and SFA laser angioplasty.

OPERATING ROOM EQUIPMENT

All procedures are performed in a cardiovascular operating room equipped for intraoperative arteriography with a surgical C-arm roentgenographic unit (Diagnost OP-C, International Surgical Systems) integrated with a videotape recorder and monitor for contrast injection visualization. An Eigen disk is also used to provide still images of selected arteriographic segments on a second monitor.

Recently available on the market is a new nonmetallic, carbon fiber surgical table (model 205, International Surgical Systems) developed especially for vascular laser procedures. The table (Fig. 9–1), supported by pedestals at either end, provides complete clearance beneath, allows 15° side-to-side roll with 20° Trendelenburg tilt (standard and reverse). A metric ruler (USA

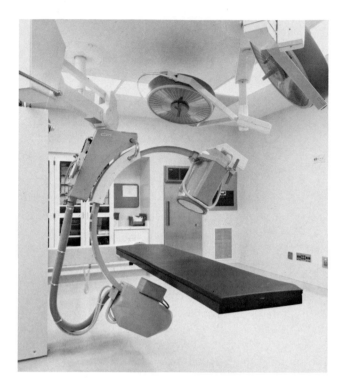

Fig. 9–1. Nonmetallic carbon fiber surgical table developed especially for vascular laser procedures has complete clearance beneath for intraoperative arteriography.

XRAY) is placed on the table beneath the patient's limb, calibrated from the level of the umbilicus, to provide reference measurements.

Laser energy is provided by an Nd:YAG source (Optilase 1000, Trimedyne, Inc.) capable of producing up to 60 W of pulsed or continuous wave energy. This has replaced the argon system in our facility because the broader performance characteristics of the Nd:YAG are compatible with probes up to 5.0 mm in diameter. However, the argon produces equally satisfactory results with probes up to 2.5 mm OD. (Newer versions of argon lasers with incrementally sized probes are undergoing clinical trials).

The laser energy is delivered through a variety of fiberoptic probes (Fig. 9–2). The most common peripheral model we use is a 2.5 mm metal-tipped probe (Laserprobe-SLR™, Trimedyne, Inc.) with a 600-μm fiber that achieves a temperature of 1,004°C in air but approximately 500°C intraluminally.

A comparably sized probe has a channel placed eccentrically on the side of the probe's tip (Laserprobe-PLR™ Flex, Trimedyne, Inc.) for passage over a 0.035 in. guidewire. This probe is employed whenever a wire has been used to cross the lesion initially, allowing lasing to be accomplished over the wire. Smaller 2.0 mm versions of these models are also available.

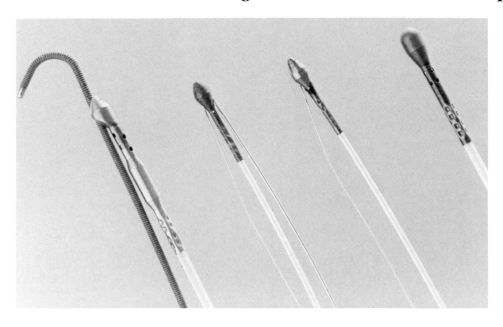

Fig. 9–2. A variety of probes are currently available for peripheral angioplasty: from left, the 2.5 mm eccentric probe (PLR-Flex) over a guidewire; two models of the 2.0 mm vascular probes (PLR-Flex and PLR-Plus); and the commonly used 2.5 mm surgical recanalization probe (SLR).

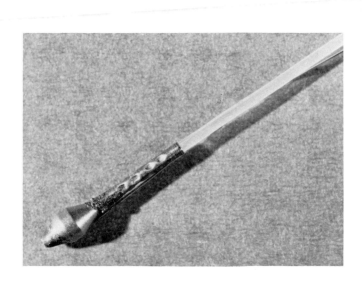

Fig. 9–3. The 2.5 mm Spectraprobe with a central opening that emits 10–20% active laser light.

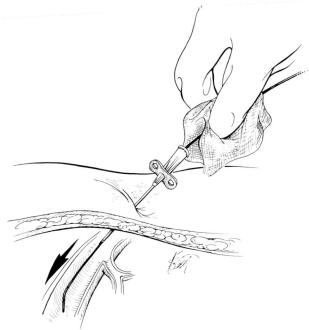

Fig. 9–4. Using a moistened gauze to hold the "eel" guidewire assists in the delivery of this extremely slippery wire.

A newer addition to the family of probes is the 2.5 mm Spectraprobe™ (Fig. 9–3) (Trimedyne, Inc.), which has a spearheaded sapphire tip with a 2 μm central window that emits 10–20% direct laser light. This probe's partial open beam preceding the metal tip appears promising in dealing with calcified lesions resistant to the closed-beam delivery system.

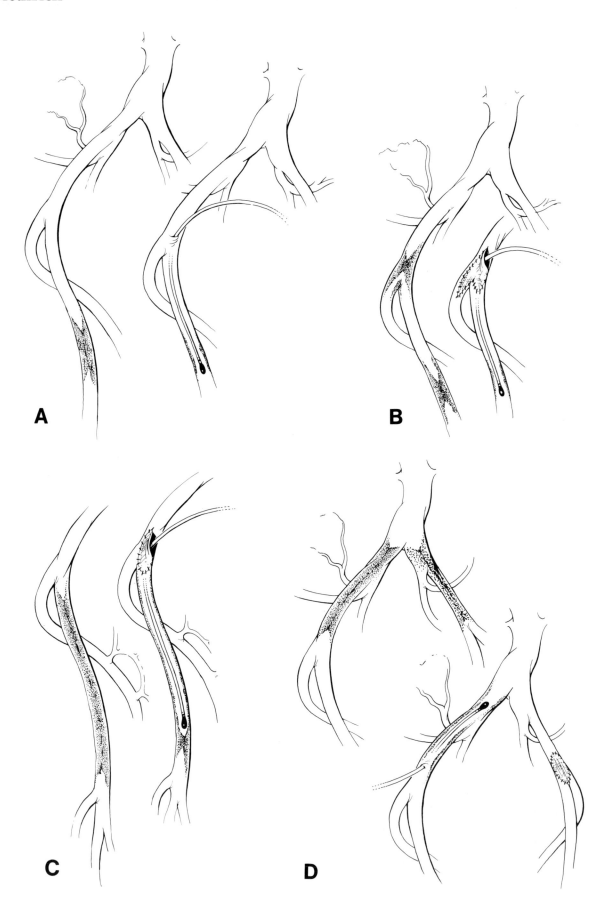

A

B

C

D

Fig. 9–5, A–D

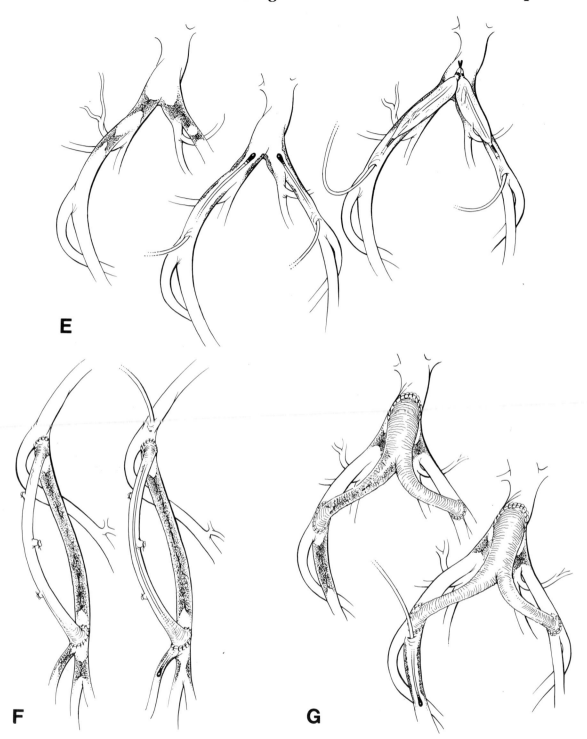

Fig. 9–5. Typical patterns of peripheral occlusive disease and laser-assisted operative techniques for revascularization. **A,** Occlusion of the SFA at the adductor hiatus (left) with percutaneous laser/balloon angioplasty (right). **B,** Common femoral and profunda femoris lesions in conjunction with superficial femoral artery disease (left). Endarterectomy (right) of the proximal lesions facilitates distal laser/balloon angioplasty of the SFA; a Dacron patch closes the arteriotomy. **C,** Total occlusion of the SFA with no proximal open segments (left). Open end arterectomy (right) and laser/balloon angioplasty of the SFA with Dacron patch grafting at the laser entry site to prevent reocclusion. **D,** Occlusion of the common and external iliac arteries (left). Even in the absence of a femoral pulse, percutaneous laser angioplasty is attempted (left side of right drawing). Should it fail, open arteriotomy is performed (represented on right branch of lower drawing); a Dacron patch graft is placed at the arteriotomy site. **E,** Bilateral iliac lesions with open common femoral artery segments (left). Each artery is lased independently, either using percutaneous or open approach (middle). Following lasing (right), the bilateral iliac lesions are dilated with simultaneous balloon inflation. **F,** Patent femoral-popliteal bypass graft compromised by distal occlusive disease (left). Laser probe is passed percutaneously through the bypass graft (right), into the infrapopliteal arteries, where the anterior tibial stenosis is lased; balloon dilatation is optional. **G,** Occluded aortofemoral bypass graft requiring reoperation with an occluded SFA (left). The graft is opened (right), and the SFA undergoes laser/balloon angioplasty. From Vascular Surgery, The Journal of Vascular Diseases, Volume 22:77–89, 1988. Reproduced with permission of the copyright owner; Westminster Publications, Inc., Roslyn, New York (U.S.A.). All rights reserved.

An 18-gauge Potts-Cournard needle with obturator (USCI-Bard) is used for the percutaneous technique. In both the percutaneous and open surgical procedures, 8 or 9 F introducers with sheaths (Cordis) are generally utilized; however, when larger arteries are encountered, 11 F or 12 F introducers may be necessary for use with the 3.5 mm probes.

Guidance is provided by a new hydrophilic, 145 cm, 0.035 in. guidewire (Glidewire, Medi-tech, Inc.) [24]. This wire becomes uncommonly slippery when wet (hence, its nickname: the "eel") and is best handled with moistened gauze (Fig. 9–4). However, it is this lubricity that makes it extremely effective in negotiating even the most severely stenosed lesions.

One precaution should be taken with this wire because of its potential heat liability: The manufacturer does not recommend its use with a heated probe, but we have averted any difficulty by simultaneously moving the probe and wire independently so that the metal tip is not in contact with any one point of the wire for a prolonged period of time.

For postlasing dilatation, a variety of balloon catheters are employed, depending on the nature of the lesions. In the SFA and popliteal arteries, the most frequently used balloons are 4, 5, or 6 mm × 10 cm (Medi-tech, Inc.); the iliac arteries require the 8 or 10 mm × 10 cm model.

PATIENT PREPARATION AND APPROACH SELECTION

Epidural block is our preferred form of anesthesia for laser-assisted procedures regardless of the entry technique. This mode of anesthesia has several advantages over local or general methods. The patient is conscious and can observe the procedure while experiencing no discomfort from the laser probe, balloon catheter, or contrast material. More importantly, though, the epidural block produces a profound sympathetic response that eliminates to a great extent the vasospasm observed with local anesthesia.

Of course, if epidural block is contraindicated (patients with previous spinal operations or in whom a thrombolytic agent will be used), local or, more rarely, general anesthesia may be employed.

Initially in our experience, bilateral SFA angioplasties were performed simultaneously. However, these procedures are now staged, doing each limb on successive days with the epidural catheter left in place while the patient stays in the intensive care unit. Patients with both iliac and SFA lesions are treated similarly, with the upper segment done initially followed by the lower lesions on the next day.

The operative approach is determined by the location of the lesions and the necessity for exposure of the common femoral artery. Since the initiation of our program, we have used the percutaneous route whenever possible, and it predominants in the approach to iliac, mid-SFA, and popliteal lesions. Figure 9–5 depicts some of the commonly observed disease configurations that are encountered and typical recanalization techniques. (These pathologies also have a role in the categorization system we have devised to predict laser success.)

In general, the open technique is required for approach to the common femoral, profunda femoris, and superficial femoral arteries in instances of 1) complete occlusion of the common or external iliac artery (with absent femoral pulse) if percutaneous needle insertion is not possible (Fig. 9–5D); 2) common femoral or profunda femoris lesions in conjunction with SFA occlusion and stenoses (Fig. 9–5B); or 3) extensive atherosclerotic disease preventing introduction of the sheath at the site of percutaneous entry.

The patient's groin is prepped in the standard manner and covered with a steridrape without any metal clips around the leg.

OPERATIVE PROCEDURES

The following are descriptions of the techniques developed for percutaneous or open access to lesions lying in the common or superficial femoral arteries and distal branches. Special procedures to be employed for iliac arterial recanalization are discussed separately.

Percutaneous Approach

Once satisfactory anesthesia is confirmed, the 18-gauge Potts-Cournard needle is introduced antegrade at the site of the femoral pulse. If the pulse cannot be palpated, the CFA is located fluoroscopically as it passes over the head of the femur by comparison with the preoperative arteriogram. Under fluoroscopic control, the tip of the needle is placed directly over the artery and inserted. When backflow substantiates access to the artery, the 0.035 in. guidewire is passed through the needle to the SFA and advanced as far as possible. With the needle removed, the appropriately sized introducer sheath is positioned in the common and proximal superficial femoral arteries. A small bolus of contrast material (Omnipaque 300, Winthrop Laboratories) is injected through the sheath to confirm its location and identify the most proximal arterial obstruction. Following sheath placement, 2,500 U of heparin sodium are administered intravenously.

With the artery thus prepared for lasing, the 2.5 mm fiberoptic probe is tested prior to use by submersion in saline to confirm the presence of energy at the tip (bubbles). With the laser turned off, the probe is passed through the sheath to the proximal lesion.

Lasing begins at 12 W with the probe constantly moving in a to-and-fro motion (this keeps the probe from sticking to the vessel wall and accumulating charred debris on the tip). Continuous contrast injection is maintained throughout lasing to monitor the probe's movement in relation to the artery, helping to avoid perforation.

Lasing is continued until the probe either creates an open channel in a total obstruction or "debulks" a tight stenosis. If long occlusions or multiple stenotic segments are found in tandem, treatment continues in stepwise fashion until all lesions have been treated. The probe is withdrawn under continuous activation so that the tip exits the sheath clean without carbon particles. With the artery opened, retrograde blood flow is observed through the sheath's side tubing.

Because the largest-sized probes available at this time cannot completely recanalize an artery in most cases, balloon dilatation is necessary to fully expand the vessel. A balloon catheter compatible with the size of the artery is introduced over the guidewire and inflated for 30 s intervals in serial fashion at each stenotic segment. If the inflation characteristics of the balloon indicate substantial residual plaque, the compromised segment is released.

Following successful dilatation, a final control arteriogram is taken before the treated arteries are released to smooth the intima. This "glazing," performed at the 12 W treatment energy setting, presumably benefits long-term patency by reducing surface irregularities to give a more satisfactory blood–intima interface.[1]

With the procedure now complete, heparinization is not reversed, and the patient is transferred to the recovery room with the sheath in place. Removal of the sheath takes place after the activated coagulation time (ACT) has fallen below 150 s.

Open Technique

Used whenever the needle cannot be placed percutaneously, the open approach begins with a vertical incision exposing the CFA from the inguinal ligament distally to its bifurcation into the origin of the profunda femoris artery and the proximal SFA. Twenty-five

hundred units of heparin are given intravenously prior to clamping the common femoral and profunda femoris arteries. In the open technique, there is often no need to clamp the SFA since it is generally occluded at its origin.

With the arteries cross-clamped, an arteriotomy is made in the CFA for introduction of the laser probe. The incision is extended approximately 3 mm into the SFA. If a significant obstruction exists in either the profunda femoris or common femoral arteries, a classical endarterectomy is performed, intentionally terminating near the origin of the SFA.

The probe is introduced and passed distally to create a 2 cm channel in the SFA. The catheter sheath is then inserted through the arteriotomy for use in further lasing, balloon dilatation, and contrast injection. The procedure continues as described in the percutaneous technique, with concomitant lesions lased and dilated sequentially.

Once all lesions are treated, the arteriotomy in the CFA is closed with a knitted Dacron patch. If a profunda endarterectomy has been performed, the patch on the CFA is extended to the profunda femoris artery as well.

It is important to note here that a flap of atherosclerotic plaque is usually created by the probe at the proximal aspect of significant SFA lesions. When opening the severely diseased SFA, the probe has a tendency to deviate posteriorly from the coaxial plane, leaving residual plaque on the anterior wall at the site of the incision (Fig. 9–6). If this flap is left untreated, the reestablished blood flow will dissect this area, causing the proximal artery to reocclude.

To prevent this problem, a new procedure has been devised, named the "boat-dock technique" (Fig. 9–7). A small piece of knitted Dacron graft material (Sauvage) is cut the length of the arteriotomy. Each end of the patch is trimmed to a point resembling the bow of a boat. The residual atherosclerotic plaque at the proximal SFA is secured anteriorly against the artery wall with 5-0 prolene suture. The Dacron patch is then sutured to the secured plaque as if a boat were being moored to a dock. When this suturing procedure is complete, the atherosclerotic plaque, like a pennant on the bow, is fixed in position. Just prior to completion of the suture line, the clamp in the SFA is released and retrograde flow from the newly created posterior channel can be observed. Attention to these details is extremely important to assure success in treating disease at the origin of the SFA.

POSTOPERATIVE TREATMENT

Patients are observed in the intensive care unit overnight for signs of bleeding or a change in pulse status.

---

[1]Editor's note: To date, there is no evidence that use of a 2.0 or 2.5 mm laser probe after balloon dilatation to 4–6 mm offers any benefit. In fact, experimental studies suggest that this technique may actually increase the risk of perforation.

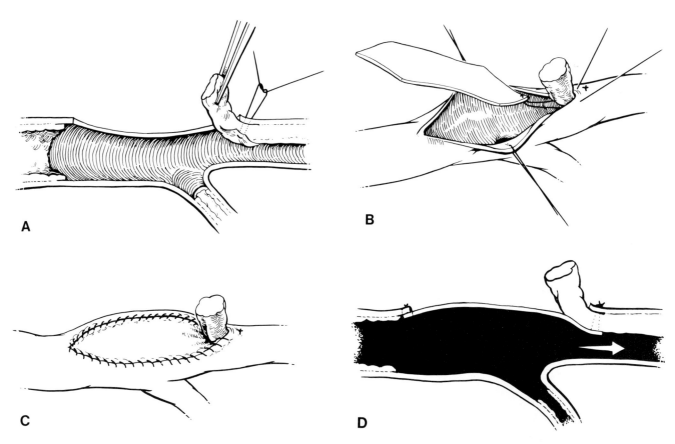

Fig. 9–6. **A,** In the open approach to severe SFA lesions, the probe encounters the plaque in the coaxial plane. **B,** However, posterior deviation of the probe creates an anterior atherosclerotic flap that, if unrepaired, can compromise circulation and cause restenosis.

Fig. 9–7. The "boat-dock" technique for anterior flap repair. **A,** The flap is secured anteriorly against the artery wall with 5-0 prolene suture. **B,** A knitted Dacron patch sized to fit the arteriotomy is trimmed to a point on either end, resembling the bow of a boat. It is moved into position over the arteriotomy as if a boat were being moored into dock. **C,** The graft is sutured in place, leaving the atherosclerotic flap exteriorized, dangling like a pennant on the boat. **D,** The flap is fixed in position to allow an unobstructed channel.

Heparin administration (1,000 cc/h IV drip) is begun 1 h after sheath removal to maintain the ACT above 200 s for 48 h. This has helped to lessen early thrombosis, and it has not caused an increase in hematoma formation at the incision site. Ambulation is begun within 12 h after the procedure, provided that are no contraindications and the recovery from anesthesia is complete.

In addition to this, the aspirin (325 mg/day) and dipyridamole (75 mg t.i.d. p.o.) begun prior to operation are reinstituted as soon as oral intake of food can be

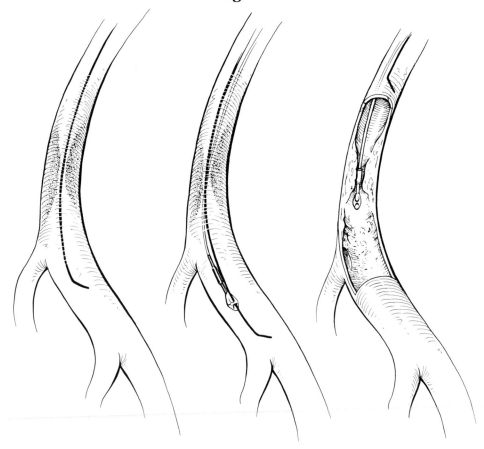

Fig. 9–8.   Reverse lasing technique for calcified lesions. The partial beam Spectraprobe creates a small channel in the plaque through which a guidewire is threaded for passage of the eccentric probe. With the wire pulled back, the probe is activated and pulled retrograde through the plaque.

tolerated. Discharge from the hospital usually takes place 1–2 days after operation.

Follow-up evaluation and exercise arterial Doppler examination is performed within 10 days. Selective arteriography and Doppler studies are scheduled at 6-month intervals for documentation of long-term results. Return of symptoms or failure to improve are indications for earlier arteriographic studies.

RESISTANT LESIONS AND RETROGRADE LASING

In cases of severe calcification, the closed beam probe may not traverse the lesion. For these cases, the new partial open beam Spectraprobe is passed to the resistant plaque and activated in the continuous mode at an energy setting of 12 W in order to open the artery with the combined efforts of the heated tip and active laser light. This probe has been effective in approximately 80% of the calcified lesions on which it has been used.

In some instances, the preceding laser light opens only a small channel through the lesion without actual penetration by the tip. Because this nonguided probe cannot be forced into a lesion for fear of deviation and perforation, a technique for reverse direction lasing is used (Fig. 9–8), in which the eccentric probe is passed through the narrow channel over a guidewire to the distal aspect of the obstruction. With the wire retracted, the probe is activated and pulled retrograde through the lesion to further open the artery.

ILIAC ARTERY RECANALIZATION

Lesions in the iliac arteries can be approached either percutaneously or surgically, depending on the disease severity at the CFA. For example, the percutaneous approach cannot be used if the external iliac artery is not open wide enough to accommodate the sheath. Furthermore, a few alterations in the technique have been developed.

Because of the larger size of these arteries, there is a greater discrepancy between the 2.5 mm probe

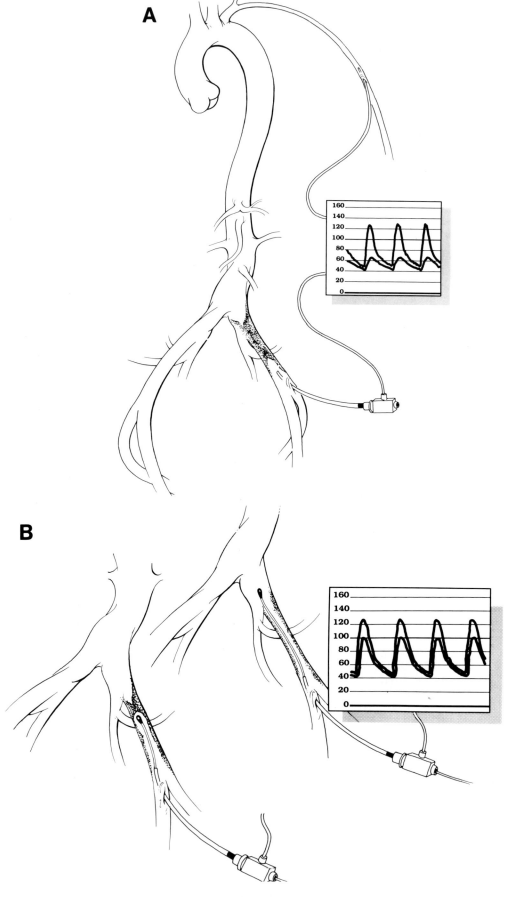

Fig. 9–9, A–B

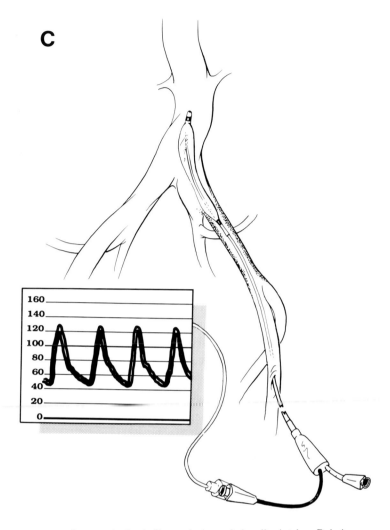

Fig. 9–9.   Pressure gradient monitoring in iliac angioplasty. **A,** baseline is taken; **B,** lasing opens a channel, but the gradient persists due to residual plaque; **C,** the segment is dilated until the gradient is abolished.

diameter and that of the artery. With a greater proportion of plaque for the balloon to displace, it is likely that the fractures and crevices produced in the plaque will be more pronounced and detrimental to uninterrupted blood flow. At this time, probes up to 5.0 mm are being evaluated in the iliac arteries; they should offer much better ablation in the larger bore arteries.

Another consideration that has added impact in the iliac arterial system is the reliability of the fluoroscopic images used to document satisfactory dilatation. Arteriograms provide information in a planar view, and reconstriction, inadequate dilatation, or an elevated intimal flap may go undetected.

To help corroborate arteriographic data and provide a positive definition for procedural success, pressure gradients are now routinely measured during iliac artery angioplasty. Attachment of a pressure line to the side

port of the sheath makes it possible to monitor the pressure gradient across the lesion (Fig. 9–9). Only when the gradient has been obliterated can the arterial segment be considered adequately recanalized.

Elimination of the pressure gradient is the single most important determinant of a successful procedure in the aortoiliac arterial segment, but even then restenosis cannot be assured. In our early experience, three patients demonstrated pulse diminution shortly after laser angioplasty. In each, it was found that the pressure gradient had not been abolished. Today, if a gradient of more than 15 mm Hg persists, or if the arterial segment appears diffusely diseased or irregular, an intravascular stent is inserted over a balloon [25,26]. The results of this technique to date have been very gratifying.

Another technical procedure useful in treating bifurcation disease is the "kissing-balloon" technique commonly used by radiologists. For bilateral disease, identical procedures are performed on both vessels. After each artery is successfully dilated, a guidewire is threaded through each into the aorta (Fig. 9–5E). Two balloons, inserted so as to lie at the bifurcation, are dilated simultaneously. This places more consistent pressure on the atherosclerotic plaque and stabilizes the bifurcation, eliminating the shifting of material from one side to the other. If both lesions are resistant to initial lasing efforts, the reverse lasing technique can also be used with dual eccentric probes.

The kissing-balloon technique is likewise applicable to the popliteal trifurcation but with the simultaneous dilatations over dual wires performed sequentially at each branching.

COMPLICATIONS

Because laser-assisted angioplasty is a relatively new technique, the definition and enumeration of complications have been from the morbidity seen in animal studies and a few low-volume clinical series that have reached publication [5,7,8,27–33].

Two of the most commonly referenced consequences of the procedure, perforation and aneurysm formation, are, in our experience, quite different from descriptions in the literature. For instance, there has been no occurrence of aneurysmal formation at a lasing site in any of our 770 procedures performed over 16 months.

In the same fashion, perforation, which has been reported to have an incidence ranging from 0 to 66% [1,2,8,13,30,34], has a rate of 7% in our cases. Part of this discrepancy may relate to the imprecise definition of perforation.

Based on our clinical experience, there have been five types of arterial injury observed that can be arranged into three categories to more accurately describe probe deviation and its effect on outcome. The injuries run from the simplest form of dissection to the most deleterious type of adventitial rupture, but only three ramifications are clinically relevant.

Class I

This category encompasses dissections that do not penetrate the adventitia. In the first scenario, the laser probe leaves the true lumen or the intended plane of dissection, deviating into an aberrant pathway. It may shear an arterial side branch, but it eventually relocates distally in the correct, open arterial channel (Fig. 9–10A). There is no adverse reaction to this dissection and, in most cases, the situation goes unnoticed.

A more consequential event is the laser probe deviating into the atherosclerotic plaque, usually when it encounters calcium deposits. Unlike the clinically sat-

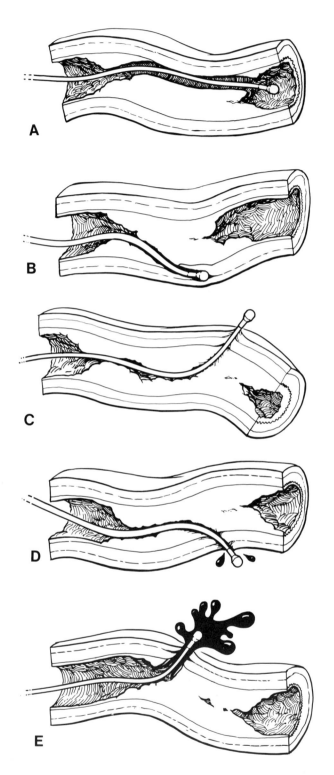

Fig. 9–10. Classification of arterial damage due to the laser probe. **A,** Class I: probe dissects from the coaxial plane but reenters the lumen, providing an adequate channel. **B,** Class I: the probe dissects the plaque or intima and does not relocate in the true lumen or restore arterial continuity; the procedure is abandoned without consequence. **C,** Class II. True adventitial wall rupture with extravasation of contrast material but no bleeding; no sequelae. **D,** Class II: Same injury as in C but blood seeps from the perforation at the site of dense plaque; clot formation seals the wound without need for surgical repair. **E,** Class III: Adventitial wall perforation with hemorrhage requiring surgical intervention.

isfactory situation above, however, the probe does not reenter the true distal lumen or create a satisfactory dissection plane that can restore arterial continuity (Fig. 9–10B). Under these circumstances, the procedure must usually be abandoned with no untoward consequences.

Class II

In this situation there is true arterial wall penetration through the adventitia (Fig. 9–10C) with two possible outcomes. In the first, contrast material may be seen outside the arterial wall, but without active bleeding. Here, in the more common situation, the probe has penetrated the artery in an area of dense atherosclerotic material, so little if any blood is flowing through that segment.

Occasionally, such an injury may be attended by leakage of blood from the artery. Because of the severe disease, the blood flow is under very low pressure, so clot formation seals the penetration site (Fig. 9–10D). No operative intervention is required, but the procedure is terminated, heparinization is reversed, and the patient is observed for any complications resulting from the perforation.

Class III

This is the same type of damage as in class II, but the active bleeding continues through the perforation site and surgical intervention is required to control the hemorrhage (Fig. 9–10E).[2]

There has been no class III perforation in our experience. Among the remaining two classes, class I injuries are slightly more common (30, 4%; class II: 24, 3%).

Preventing perforation depends to a large extent on the operator's skills in sensing resistance to the probe's advances and localization of the tip's relative position in the artery using contrast material. Knowing when and how to use the partial beam probe can make a significant difference in perforation rates.

Vasospasm is another intraoperative complication that may be encountered. It is infrequent in our experience (< 1%) due to the epidural anesthesia, but it can be treated with intraarterial papaverine (60 mg) to relieve the constriction.

Thrombosis is primarily a postoperative problem (although there was one incident intraoperatively in our series when heparinization was inadvertently overlooked with resultant acute thrombosis). The damage inflicted on the intima and plaque by the combined lasing and dilating techniques can encourage platelet aggregation and fibrin deposition. Arterial wall collapse of the dilated segment has also been implicated in thrombus formation.

Acute thrombosis should be documented by arteriography and then treated with 250,000 U of urokinase injected as a loading dose through a catheter positioned at the clot. Infusion continues at 4,000 U/min with repeat arteriographic studies to confirm clot lysis. Relasing after the clot has been lysed has often been successful, but intravascular stenting should be considered if the artery fails to retain its lumen after dilatation.

The puncture site can be a source of difficulty. Hematoma formation was common early in our experience, but only rarely did it require evacuation. It is now routine for pressure to be applied to the wound for 30 min after sheath removal to assist with clotting. False aneurysms at the puncture site were seen occasionally after sheath removal in hypertensive patients whose blood pressure was elevated. Good hemostatic control can avoid this problem.

DISEASE/SEGMENT CATEGORIZATION AND LASER SUCCESS

During the evolution of our techniques, it became obvious that outcome was related to the location, nature, and extent of the atherosclerotic disease process. Table 9–1 presents the arterial distribution of the 770 lesions lased in 400 patients over a 16-month period at the Arizona Heart Institute.

Overall, in this 16-month experience, either the pulse was restored or Doppler studies showed improvement postoperatively in 580 (75%) procedures. Of the 190 failed procedures, 42 (22%) were due to calcification blocking probe penetration, 20 (11%) resulted from poor distal runoff, 38 (20%) thrombosed and were repeated, and 54 (28%) suffered perforations requiring conversion to standard bypass grafting. The remaining 36 (19%) saw no improvement for reasons as yet undetermined.

By category, the best results were seen in the SFA segment, surprisingly with slightly better outcome in the occluded vessels at the mid-artery level. Results in the popliteal segment were comparable. Tibial/peroneal lesions faired worst of all, although these are short-term results that may change during the follow-up evaluations now in progress.

---

[2]Editor's note: Intraarterial balloon tamponade can also be used to control and, in most cases, stop the bleeding without the need for surgical repair.

TABLE 9–1. Procedural Success for Laser Angioplasty in 400 Patients

Category	No. lesions	Laser success
I (Iliac)	133 (17%)	98 (74%)
A. Occlusion	73	44 (60%)
B. Stenosis	60	54 (90%)
II (SFA)	418 (54%)	331 (80%)
A. Occlusion		
Proximal	192	140 (73%)
Mid	73	68 (93%)
B. Occlusion/no runoff	10	2 (20%)
C. Stenosis	143	121 (85%)
III (Popliteal)	121 (16%)	96 (79%)
A. Occlusion	59	44 (75%)
B. Occlusion/no runoff	9	5 (56%)
C. Stenosis	53	47 (89%)
IV (Tibial/peroneal)	73 (9%)	45 (62%)
A. Occlusion	17	12 (71%)
B. Occlusion/no runoff	18	4 (22%)
C. Stenosis	38	29 (76%)
Grafts	25 (3%)	10 (66%)
A. Vein	12	5 (43%)
B. Prosthetic	13	11 (88%)
Totals	770 (100%)	580 (75%)

Stenotic lesions in all segments responded well except the tibial/peroneal arteries, where recanalization was slightly more successful in the occluded segments. Laser treatment of grafts was moderately successful.

THE FUTURE

The proliferation of laser delivery systems under development clearly indicates that we can expect some major improvements in the not too distant future. Incrementally sized probes have been anticipated as an answer to two problems. First, the difficulty of penetrating tight lesions, with their higher probability for perforation, should be reduced with small probes (1 mm). Using gradually increasing diameters could safely open a sufficient channel. The thinner probes would also be desirable for the smaller distal vessels.

In the larger bore arteries, graduated probes up to and beyond 5 mm would be able to open wider channels needing less balloon dilatation. Ideally, the probes could be sequentially used to establish an optimum channel without dilatation. This would obviate the balloon damage to the intima and plaque and should lessen thrombosis and restenosis.

The power behind the probes will most probably undergo significant change. The excimer laser has been eagerly awaited; it has no thermal effect, making it possible to perform precise ablative cuts in the plaque without the charring produced by the metal tip probe. However, on the other hand, the thermal effect of the closed beam probe seems to reduce surface thrombogenicity, whereas the excimer leaves the treated area as thrombogenic as it was before lasing.

All this anticipated improvement in technology will tend to keep laser-assisted angioplasty in a state of flux: it will be several years more before we can arrive at a standardized technique that can be adequately assessed for efficacy, as happened with transluminal coronary angioplasty.

For now, the use of lasers by vascular surgeons seems a logical extension of our skills. We are able to utilize the technology to its fullest capability without access limitations, giving us the perfect opportunity to broaden its applications and evaluate their effects. It is indeed a "bright" and promising auxiliary tool and well on its way toward becoming a replacement for bypass grafting in the lower extremities in many patients.

REFERENCES

1. Abela GS, Norman SJ, Cohen D, Feldman RL, Geiser EA, Conti CR: Laser recanalization of occluded atherosclerotic arteries: An in vivo and in vitro study. Circulation 71:403–411, 1985.

2. Abela GS, Seeger JM, Barbieri E, Franzini D, Fenech A, Pepine CJ, Conti CR: Laser angioplasty with angioscopic guidance in humans. J Am Coll Cardiol 8:184–192, 1986.

3. Crea F, Davies G, McKenna W, Pashazade M, Taylor K, Maseri C: Percutaneous laser recanalization of coronary arteries. (letter) Lancet 2:214, 1986.

4. Cumberland DC, Sanborn T, Taylor DI, Ryan TJ: Percutaneous laser thermal angioplasty: Clinical experience in peripheral artery occlusions. J Am Coll Cardiol 2:211A, 1986.

5. Cumberland DC, Sanborn TA, Taylor DI, Moore DJ, Welsh CL, Greenfield AJ, Guben JK, Ryan TJ: Percutaneous laser thermal angioplasty: Initial clinical results with a laser probe in total peripheral artery occlusions. Lancet 1:1457–1459, 1986.

6. Cumberland DC, Taylor DI, Proctor AE: Laser-assisted percutaneous angioplasty: Initial clinical experience in peripheral arteries. Clin Radiol 37:423–428, 1986.

7. Dries DJ, Lawrence PF, Syverud J, Moatamed F, Dixon J: Response of atherosclerotic aorta to argon laser. Lasers Surg Med 5:321–326, 1985.

8. Ginsberg R, Wexler L, Mitchell RS, Profitt D: Percutaneous transluminal laser angioplasty for treatment of peripheral vascular disease: Clinical experience with sixteen patients. Radiology 156:619–624, 1985.

9. Grundfest WS, Litvak F, Forrester JS, Goldenberg J, Swan HS, Morgenstern L, Fishbein N, McDermid IS, Rider DM, Pacala TJ: Laser ablation of human atherosclerotic plaque without adjacent tissue injury. J Am Coll Cardiol 5:929–933, 1985.

10. Grundfest WS, Litvak F, Hickey A: The current status of angioscopy and laser angioplasty. J Vasc Surg 5:667–673, 1987.

11. Kaplan MD, Case RB, Choy DS: Vascular recanalization with argon laser: Role of blood in transmission of laser energy. Lasers Surg Med 5:275–279, 1985.

12. Sanborn TA, Faxon DP, Kellett MA, Ryan TJ: Percutaneous coronary laser thermal angioplasty. J Am Coll Cardiol 8:1437–1440, 1986.

13. Sanborn TA, Greenfield AJ, Guben JK, Menzoian JO, LoGerfo FW: Human percutaneous and intraoperative laser thermal angioplasty: Initial clinical results as an adjunct to balloon angioplasty. J Vasc Surg 5:83–90, 1987.

14. Selzer DM, Murphy-Chutporan D, Ginsburg R, Wexler L: Optimizing strategies for laser angioplasty. Invest Radiol 20:860–866, 1985.

15. Diethrich EB, Kinard SA, Webb GE, Scappatura E, Mitsuoka H, Moiel D: Intraoperative coronary arteriography. Am J Surg 124:815–818, 1972.

16. Diethrich EB, Kinard SA: Coronary arteriography in the operating room. Medicamundi 19:12–19, 1974.

17. Diethrich EB: Intraoperative coronary arteriography: A predictor of graft patency. Medicamundi 23:107–111, 1978.

18. Diethrich EB, Rozaci J, Timbadia E, Bahadir I, Coburn K, Zenzen S: Laser angioplasty—A surgical perspective. Medicamundi 32:127–132, 1987.

19. Diethrich EB, Rozaci J, Timbadia E, Bahadir I, Coburn K, Zenzen S: Argon laser-assisted peripheral angioplasty. Vasc Surg 22:77–87, 1988.

20. Diethrich EB, Timbadia E, Bahadir I: Applications and limitations of laser-assisted angioplasty. Eur J Vasc Surg 3: 12–21, 1989.

21. Diethrich EB, Timbadia E, Bahadir I, Carroll S, Zenzen S, Coburn S: Intraoperative coronary laser recanalization: evaluation of safety in ten patients. Vasc Surg 22: 335–343, 1988.

22. Diethrich EB, Timbadia E, Bahadir I: Peripheral laser-assisted angioplasty. In Montorsi W (ed): Proceedings of the XXVI World Congress of the International College of Surgeons. Milan, Italy: Monduzzi Editore, 1988 pp 433–436.

23. Diethrich EB, Timbadia E, Bahadir I: Peripheral laser angioplasty. In Muller GJ, Biamino G (eds): Advances in Laser Medicine I: First German Symposium on Laser Angioplasty. Berlin: Ecomed Verlagsgesellschaft, 1988: 217–226.

24. Diethrich EB, Timbadia E, Bahadir I: Hydrophilic guidewire for laser-assisted angioplasty (letter). J Vasc Surg 8: 201–202, 1988.

25. Sigwart U, Puel J, Mirkovitch V, Joffre F, Kappenberger L: Intravascular stents to prevent occlusion and restenosis after transluminal angioplasty. N Engl J Med 316:701–706, 1987.

26. Schatz RA, Palmaz JL: Intravascular stents for angioplasty. Cardiology 12:27–31, 1987.

27. Isner JM, Donaldson RF, Funai JT, Deckelbaum LI, Randian NG, Clarke RH, Konstam MA, Salem DN, Bernstein JS: Factors contributing to perforations resulting from laser coronary angioplasty: Observations in an intact human postmortem preparation of intraoperative laser coronary angioplasty. Circulation (Suppl II) 72:II-191–199, 1985.

28. Labs JD, Merillat JC, Williams GM: Analysis of solid phase debris from laser angioplasty: Potential risks of atheroembolism. J Vasc Surg 7:326–335, 1988.

29. Choy DS, Stertzer S, Loubeau JM, Kesseler H, Quilici P, Rotterdam H, Meltzer L: Embolization and vessel wall perforation in argon laser recanalization. Lasers Surg Med 5:297–308, 1985.

30. Sanborn TA, Faxon DP, Haudenschild C, Ryan TJ: Experimental angioplasty: Circumferential distribution of laser thermal energy with a laser probe. J Am Coll Cardiol 5:934–945, 1985.

31. Lee G, Ikeda RM, Theis JH, Chan MC, Stobbe D, Ogata C, Kumagai A, Mason DT: Acute and chronic complications of laser angioplasty: Vascular wall damage and formation of aneurysms in the atherosclerotic rabbit. Am J Cardiol 53:290–293, 1984.

32. Lee G, Ikeda RM, Chan MC, Lee MH, Rink JL, Reis RL, Theis JH, Low R, Bommer WJ, Kung AH, Hanna ES, Mason DT: Limitations, risks and complications of laser recanalization: A cautious approach warranted. Am J Cardiol 56:181–185, 1985.

33. Cumberland DC, Tayler DI, Procter AE: Percutaneous laser angioplasty. Initial clinical experience. Ann Radiol (Paris) 29:215–218, 1986.

34. Sanborn TA, Haudenschild CC, Garber GR, Ryan TJ, Faxon DP: Angiographic and histologic consequences of laser thermal angioplasty: Comparison with balloon angioplasty. Circulation 75:1281–1286, 1987.

10. One-Year Follow-Up Results for Femoropopliteal Lesions Treated With Laser-Assisted Balloon Angioplasty

Timothy A. Sanborn, M.D.

EXPERIMENTAL AND CLINICAL BACKGROUND

Initial clinical experience with 1.5 mm and 2.0 mm diameter laser probes [1,2] indicate their safety and efficacy as an adjunct to conventional peripheral balloon angioplasty. In addition, it was reported that laser thermal angioplasty has the potential to increase the number of patients suitable for angioplasty by safely recanalizing lesions that could not be treated by conventional means [1]. Until recently, however, the long-term consequences of laser-assisted balloon angioplasty were unknown.

Theoretically, there was concern that thermal injury to the vessel wall could promote thrombosis or accelerate atherosclerosis. However, in experimental studies in atherosclerotic rabbits, this was not found to be the case [3]. In fact, in a comparative study, lesions treated with laser thermal angioplasty actually had less angiographic restenosis and significantly larger lumens than those lesions treated with conventional balloon angioplasty. On histology, 4 weeks after the laser procedure, there was a larger lumen, minimal thrombosis or smooth muscle cell proliferation, and a thin neointima covered with a fibrous cap. In contrast, those vessels treated with balloon angioplasty demonstrate evidence of prior fracture and dissection of the vessel wall [4] with more of a fibrocellular proliferative response and ongoing thrombus formation. Morphometric analysis of these histologic cross sections confirmed a significantly larger luminal area after laser thermal angioplasty compared with balloon angioplasty.

Thus, laser thermal angioplasty was associated with less restenosis and produced a significantly larger lumen compared with conventional balloon angioplasty. The differences in the pathophysiology of these techniques is probably responsible for these observations;

that is, with laser recanalization of these high-grade stenotic lesions, there is 1) partial laser vaporization or removal of atherosclerotic material and 2), perhaps more importantly, a smoother, less thrombogenic surface is left behind compared with balloon angioplasty. Whether there is an additional thermal effect on the arterial wall that inhibits platelet accumulation and/or smooth muscle cell proliferation is another intriguing concept.

These results in cholesterol-fed rabbits with balloon deendothelialized vessels are encouraging; however, the key question that remains is whether laser angioplasty can reduce restenosis clinically. At present, the laser-probe device is the only laser delivery system with adequate clinical experience for assessment of long-term results. In addition, because of the limited size of these devices (1.5 and 2.0 mm), subsequent balloon angioplasty was always required in large 5–6 mm peripheral vessels. Thus, to date, clinical data exist only on laser-assisted balloon angioplasty. However, these initial results do suggest that lasers may have an effect on restenosis and provide the stimulus for additional laser catheter development as well as further experimental and clinical studies of the use of lasers for prevention of restenosis. The following is a summary of the recently published one-year follow-up results from Boston University Medical Center and Northern General Hospital for laser-assisted balloon angioplasty of femoropopliteal stenoses and occlusion [5].

PATIENT SELECTION

Between April 1985 and December 1986, laser thermal angioplasty was performed in 129 femoropopliteal arteries in 119 patients as an adjunct to conventional balloon angioplasty. In this initial feasibility series, in order to determine the utility of this technique, laser-assisted balloon angioplasty was performed in all patients referred for femoropopliteal artery angioplasty except in those patients with short straightforward stenoses easily treated with conven-

Laser Angioplasty, pages 93–99

TABLE 10–1. Angiographic and Clinical Success

Lesion	Number	Angiographic success	Clinical success
Stenosis			
1–3 cm	14	14 (100)	14 (100)
4–7 cm	3	3 (100)	3 (100)
>7 cm	5	5 (100)	4 (80)
Total	22	22 (100)	21 (95)
Occlusion			
1–3 cm	17	17 (100)	17 (100)
4–7 cm	37	31 (84)	26 (70)
>7 cm	53	43 (81)	35 (66)
Total	107	91 (85)	78 (72)

Numbers in parentheses represent percent success in each group.

tional balloon angioplasty or atherectomy. The presence of calcium in the lesions was not an exclusion criterium. The type and length of lesions treated is summarized in Table 10–1. Diabetes mellitus was present in 16% of the patients, and 69% of the patients gave a history of cigarette smoking. In 21 of these patients, a prior attempt at conventional balloon angioplasty failed. The clinical indications for angioplasty were severe claudication that was unresponsive to exercise therapy and Trental (pentoxifylline) in 66% of patients and to rest pain, nonhealing ulcer, or gangrene in 34% of patients. Initial evaluation included a history and physical examination as well as a Doppler ankle-arm index (AAI) that was also used for follow-up after angioplasty. Patients were pretreated with oral aspirin (75 or 325 mg once a day) prior to the procedure. The laser systems and percutaneous techniques used in this series are described elsewhere in this volume and in previous reports [1,2,5].

INTERPRETATION OF RESULTS

In this study, the results of laser-assisted balloon angioplasty were classified as they were in previous reports in the radiology literature [6–8] in the manner described in the paragraphs that follow.

Angiographic and Clinical Success

This was defined as an angiographic improvement in the luminal diameter to less than 50% residual stenosis, relief of symptoms, improved pulse, and an increase in the Doppler AAI by greater than 0.15, as previously described [6–8].

Angiographic Success but Immediate Clinical Failure

In this group, some improvement in the angiographic luminal diameter was observed; however, the angiographic appearance was less than ideal (small luminal diameter, significant luminal irregularities). Symptoms were not relieved and the Doppler AAI did not increase. As in other studies [6–8], patients in this category were excluded from calculation of long-term results.

Angiographic Failure

Inability to cross the lesion with the laser-probe device or to improve the appearance of the lesion less than 50% residual stenosis was considered an angiographic (technical) failure.

Clinical Patency

All patients were followed up with periodic office visits that consisted of a careful history, physical examination, and measurements of the Doppler AAI with cumulative clinical patency determined by the life table method [9].

Recurrence

Return of the symptoms after initial clinical success was considered a recurrence, which was confirmed by repeat angiography. If symptoms returned and the patient could be successfully treated with redilation or repeat laser-assisted balloon angioplasty of a recurrent lesion, this was still considered a recurrence rather than as continued long-term patency as it was in a few other studies of conventional balloon angioplasty [6–8].

INITIAL RESULTS

Initial Success Rate: Stenoses

Of 22 femoropopliteal stenoses treated with laser-assisted balloon angioplasty, 21 (95%) had both angiographic and initial clinical success. While angiographic improvement was documented in all patients (100%), one patient with 39 cm of diffuse disease did not show clinical improvement because of thrombosis at the site of balloon angioplasty in the origin of the superficial femoral artery (Table 10–1). The mean length of stenoses for the entire group was 4.4 ± 4.1 cm (SD). The

TABLE 10–2. Complications in 129 Lesions

	No.	%
Emergency bypass surgery	0	0
Perforation	5	4.0
Dissection with probe	2	1.6
Dissection with guidewire	1	0.8
Thrombosis in first 72 h	3	2.3
Transient embolization in 24 h	1	0.8

mean AAI rose from 0.57 to 0.80 in the 21 successfully treated stenoses.

For these 22 stenoses, the 100% angiographic or technical success and 95% clinical success compares quite favorably to a recently published series of 100 stenoses treated by conventional balloon angioplasty where the technical (angiographic) success was 95.7% and the clinical success was 86.2% [7]. In another recently published series, the initial clinical success in 127 femoropopliteal stenoses was 92.2% [8]. Obviously, the present series is small and lesion characteristics and clinical situations may vary; however, there is a suggestion that laser-assisted balloon angioplasty may improve the initial success rate in stenoses. Certainly, by increasing the lumen size with laser thermal angioplasty, passage of the guidewire and advancement of the balloon angioplasty catheter through a lesion was easier.

Initial Success in Occlusions

Previously, an 89% angiographic and an 86% clinical success was reported in the first 56 total peripheral artery occlusions treated by laser thermal angioplasty as an adjunct to balloon angioplasty [1]. In the present larger series of 107 femoropopliteal occlusions, an 85% angiographic and a 73% clinical success was observed with an increase in the mean AAI from 0.63 to 0.84. This decrease in success rate is most likely due to the longer length of lesion attempted as experience and confidence was gained. In the initial series, the mean lesion length was 8 cm, whereas in the last 51 occlusions, it was 10 cm. Twenty-one of these lesions could not be treated by conventional balloon angioplasty alone. The majority of the technical and clinical failures were in lesions greater than 7 cm (19/30 or 63%), with 16 of these failures occurring in lesions greater than 10 cm.

When the occlusions were subdivided by length of lesion, the clinical success rate was 100% for short occlusions (1–3 cm), whereas lower success rates of 70 and 66% were obtained for longer lesions of 4–7 cm

and greater then 7 cm, respectively. For the 18 short occlusions, this initial success rate of 100% is higher than two recently published results for balloon angioplasty alone in which success rates for 1–3 cm occlusions were 83 [7] and 89% [6]. In the present study, the clinical success rate for occlusions greater than 3 cm was 68%. Other recent studies report clinical success rates varying from 26–78% [6–8] for occlusions greater than 3 cm; however, neither further subdivision of the lesions nor indication of the mean length of lesion were indicated in these studies. Therefore, more direct comparison is not possible.

FAILURES AND COMPLICATIONS

In the one stenosis and 29 occlusions in which both angiographic and clinical success could not be obtained, the reasons for failure were due to the following: inability in crossing lesions (n = 6), inadequate balloon dilatation (n = 8), perforation with the probe (n = 5), thrombosis in the first 24 h (n = 3), inadequate distal vessel runoff (n = 3), probe dissection (n = 2), wire dissection (n = 2), and inability to direct (steer) the probe away from a collateral vessel in one lesion. Most importantly, with this combined technique of using laser thermal angioplasty as an adjunct to balloon angioplasty 1) there was no requirement for emergency bypass surgery and 2) there was only a 4% incidence of vessel perforation. Clinically, vessel perforation was never a serious complication as it generally occurred in the hard fibrotic area at the end of a long total occlusion. The minimal contrast extravasation usually stopped within a few seconds either without additional treatment or after reversal of heparin with protamine sulfate. No significant pain, swelling, or hematoma resulted from perforation. The 4% incidence of vessel perforation with the laser probe is much lower than previous clinical series using bare argon laser fiberoptics for peripheral laser angioplasty in which vessel perforation was noted in 3 of 16 (19%) [10] and of 2 of 15 (13%) [11] vessels. In fact, the 4% perforation rate is similar to a 3% incidence of vessel perforation reported with conventional balloon angioplasty [12,13]. The incidence of other complications is not in excess of what has been reported for conventinal angioplasty [12,13]. Complication for the entire series of 129 lesions are summarized in Table 10–2.

The decreased incidence of vessel perforation with this device is probably multifactorial. From a design standpoint, the rounded but tapered tip provides a blunt object that is less likely to mechanically perforate the artery compared with sharp, pointed fiberoptics [14]. Second, the metal probe has been shown to disperse

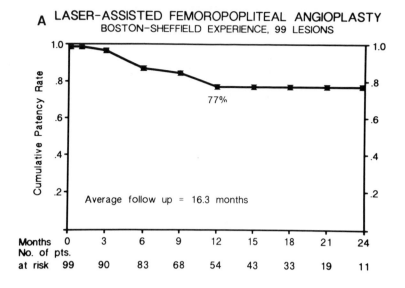

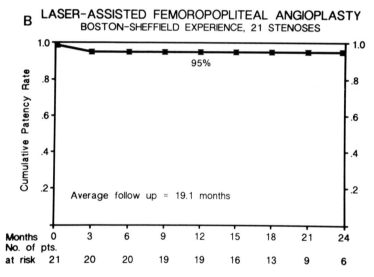

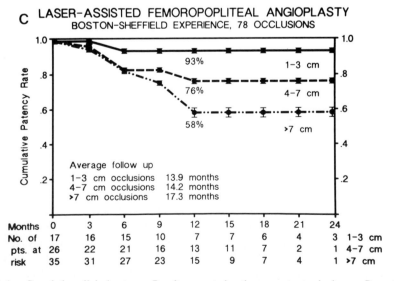

Fig. 10–1.   Cumulative clinical patency. Results presented as the mean ± standard error. Reproduced with permission of T.A. Sanborn et al. (Radiology 168:121–125, 1988).

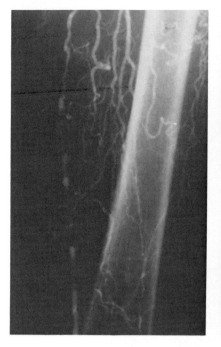 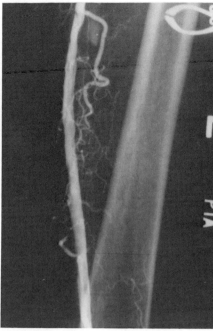 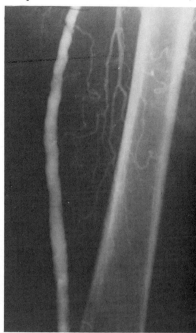

Fig. 10–2. Angiography of a 4-cm superficial femoral artery occlusion with a tortuous 8-cm stenosis proximal to the occlusion. Left panel: Prior to angioplasty. Middle panel: Immediately after laser-assisted balloon angioplasty. In this lesion, transversing the tortuous proximal stenosis required shaping a curve in the 0.014-in guidewire attached to the laser probe. The curved guidewire then provided the ability to torque the laser probe through the stenosis. After crossing the occlusion with the laser-heated probe, the probe was slowly withdrawn through the occlusion and the stenosis with the continuous laser-pulse delivery to further enlarge the entire lumen prior to balloon angioplasty. Right panel: Repeat angiography 2 months later at the time of angioplasty of the opposite leg. Reproduced with permission of T.A. Sanborn et al. (Radiology 168:121–125, 1988).

thermal energy uniformly around the tip so as not to focus all laser energy in one spot [15]. Histologic analysis after the use of this device indicates a thermal effect around the entire luminal circumference of a diseased vessel [14]. Thus, dispersion and circumferential distribution of thermal energy rather than aiming a narrow laser beam could also contribute to reduce perforation. Finally, it has been shown that vaporization and fibrofatty plaque is possible at lower temperature than it is for normal (elastic and collagen) vessel wall tissue [15]; this may also contribute to reduce perforation.

FOLLOW-UP RESULTS

Of the 99 successfully treated lesions, the overall one year cumulative clinical patency for all stenoses and occlusions was 77%. For the patients with continued clinical patency, the mean AAI on follow-up was 0.87 for the stenoses and 0.85 for occlusions compared to an index immediately postprocedure of 0.80 and 0.85, respectively. When the lesions were separated into groups, the following cumulative clinical patencies were observed: all stenoses (95%), occlusions of 1–3 cm (93%), occlusions of 4–7 cm (76%), and occlusions of greater than 7

cm (58%). These results are summarized in Figure 10–1. Angiographic examples of successful laser-assisted balloon angioplasty and follow-up arteriogram 2 and 12 months later are shown in Figures 10–2 and 10–3.

Depending on the types of lesions included in various series and the definitions of patency, the one year cumulative clinical patency rates for balloon angioplasty vary from 56 to 84% [6]. In subgroup analysis, however, a potential benefit of laser-assisted balloon angioplasty is revealed. For example, the one-year clinical patency rates for stenoses and short 1–3 cm occlusions were 95 and 93%, respectively. These results were considerably higher than recent balloon angioplasty series in which one-year patency rates were 72–81% for stenoses and 67–93% for short occlusions [7–9]. For longer occlusions, treated with laser-assisted balloon angioplasty, one-year clinical patency rates of 76% for medium-length occlusions (4–7 cm) and 58% for occlusions greater than 7 cm are also better than a patency rate of 50% for occlusions greater than 3 cm in one series [7]. The definition of clinical patency is important in comparing these results, as redilation was not considered a recurrence in two of these recent series [7,8]. In the largest of these studies [8], 26 of 129 lesions (20%) required redilation but were still included in the

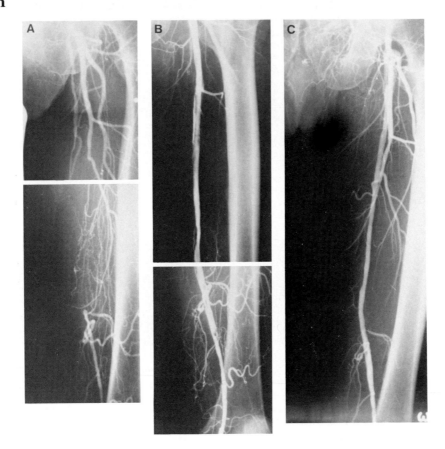

Fig. 10–3. Angiography of an 18-cm left superficial femoral artery occlusion (left panel) that was recanalized first with a 2.0 mm Laserprobe-PLR™-Plus using eight sequential pulses (5–10 s each) of 10 W of argon laser energy delivered to the probe tip. The lesion was then dilated along the entire length of the lesion with a 6 mm × 10-cm balloon catheter (middle panel). One year later, the patient was asymptomatic in his left leg, but had developed symptoms in his right leg. On diagnostic arter-

iogram, the left superficial femoral artery was still patent (right panel) and the right superficial femoral artery had a short lesion that could be treated successfully with conventional balloon angioplasty. One-year follow-up arteriogram courtesy of Dr. Gerald L. Honick, M.D., Oklahoma City, OK. Reproduced with permission of T.A. Sanborn et al. (Laser Medicine & Surgery News & Advances 6:26–35, 1988).

long-term patency group. A comparison of these 1-year patency rates is summarized in Table 10–3.

On the one hand, these initial results are influenced by the operator's learning experience and the initial development stage for this device; clinical success and patency should improve with more experience and device modifications. On the other hand, the improved follow-up results in this study compared with other recently published reports could be influenced by other patient factors, such as diabetes, smoking, distal vessel runoff, and the medications taken before and after angioplasty. Obviously, these results have to be repeated in other centers to confirm these observations. These initial results do serve as a useful reference for future laser devices.

Possible explanations for these lower recurrence rates after laser thermal angioplasty are that the technique partially removes the atherosclerotic lesion and leaves behind a smoother arterial surface. Interestingly, when recurrence was confirmed with repeat angiography, it did not always occur at the laser-treated segment, but

did recur at some point along the dilated vessel. Further angiographic analysis of the nature of recurrence after laser-assisted balloon angioplasty vs. balloon angioplasty alone would be interesting beyond this initial study. Obviously, for longer occlusions, more atherosclerotic material has to be removed, and this may be beyond the capacity of the current 2.0 mm or newer 2.5 mm laser-heated probes in 5 mm vessels. Larger probes may be beneficial in removing more material or leaving behind a smoother surface with a larger lumen so that balloon angioplasty may not be required at all. The recent study in the rabbit iliac atherosclerotic model suggests that the laser thermal angioplasty alone may cause less restenosis than does conventional balloon angioplasty alone [3].

CONCLUSIONS

This study represented the first follow-up report of this new technique of percutaneous laser thermal an-

TABLE 10–3. Comparison of 1-Year Cummulative Patency Rates

	Stenoses (%)	Occlusions		
		<3 cm (%)	4–7 cm (%)	>7 cm (%)
Laser-assisted balloon angioplasty	95	93	76	58
Balloon angioplasty alone				
Krepel et al. [6]	80	93	50 (>3 cm)	
Hewes et al. [7]	81[a]	67[a]	82[a]	68[a]
Murray et al. [8]	72[a]	86[a] (all occlusions)		

[a]12–20% redilation rate not considered a recurrence.

gioplasty used as an adjunct to balloon angioplasty in which there is a suggestion that the clinical patency for femoropopliteal lesions after laser-assisted balloon angioplasty with 1.5–2.0 mm laser probes may be greater than recent historical reports for conventional balloon angioplasty alone [5–7]. Ultimately, a randomized clinical trial comparing laser thermal angioplasty to balloon angioplasty or even bypass surgery would be in order; however, such a trial should await further improvements in the technique and the equipment (i.e., larger "over-the-wire" devices). Potentially, by improving the initial success rate and, more importantly, the long-term clinical patency, laser thermal angioplasty could improve upon the underutilization of angioplasty [16] as a non-surgical treatment of peripheral vascular disease.

REFERENCES

1. Cumberland DC, Sanborn TA, Tayler DI, Moore DJ, Welsh CL, Greenfield AJ, Guben JK, Ryan TJ: Percutaneous laser thermal angioplasty: Initial clinical results with a laserprobe in total peripheral artery occlusions. Lancet I:1457–1459, 1986.

2. Sanborn TA, Greenfield AJ, Guben JK, Menzoian JO, LoGerfo FW: Human percutaneous and intraoperative laser thermal angioplasty: Initial clinical results as an adjunct to balloon angioplasty. J Vasc Surg 5:83–90, 1987.

3. Sanborn TA, Haudenschild CC, Faxon DP, Garber GR, Ryan TJ: Angiographic and histologic consequences of laser thermal angioplasty: Comparison with balloon angioplasty. Circulation 75:281–286, 1987.

4. Sanborn TA, Faxon DP, Haudenschild CC, Gottsman SB, Ryan TJ: The mechanism of transluminal angioplasty: Evidence for formation of aneurysm in experimental atherosclerosis. Circulation 68:1136–1140, 1983.

5. Sanborn TA, Cumberland DC, Greenfield AJ, Welsh CL, Guben JK: Percutaneous laser thermal angioplasty: Initial

results and 1-year follow-up in 129 femoropopliteal lesions. Radiology 168:21–25, 1988.

6. Krepel VM, van Andel GJ, van Erp WFM, Breslau PJ: Percutaneous transluminal angioplasty of the femoropopliteal artery: Initial and long term results. Radiology 156:325–328, 1985.

7. Hewes RC, White RI, Murray RR, Kaufman SL, Chang R, Kadir S, Kinninson ML, Mitchell SE, Auster M: Long-term results of superficial femoral artery angioplasty. Am J Radiol 146:1025–1029, 1986.

8. Murray RR, Hewes RL, White RI, Mitchell SE, Auster M, Chang R, Kadir S, Kinnison ML, Kaufman SL: Long segment femoropopliteal stenoses: Is angioplasty a boom or a bust? Radiology 162:473–476, 1987.

9. Cutler SJ, Ederer F: Maximum utilization of the life table method in analyzing survival. J Chronic Dis 8:699–712, 1958.

10. Ginsburg R, Wexler L, Mitchell RS, Profitt D: Percutaneous transluminal laser angioplasty for treatment of peripheral vascular disease. Clinical experience with 16 patients. Radiology 156:619–624, 1985.

11. Cumberland DC, Tayler DI, Procter AE: Laser-assisted percutaneous angioplasty: Initial clinical experience in peripheral arteries. Clin Radiol 37:423–428, 1986.

12. Sos TA, Sniderman KW: Percutaneous transluminal angioplasty. Semin Roentgenol XVI:26–41m 1981.

13. Gardiner GA, Meyerovitz MF, Stokes KR, Clouse ME, Harrington DP, Bettmann MA: Complications of transluminal angioplasty. Radiology 159:201–208, 1986.

14. Sanborn TA, Faxon DP, Haudenschild CC, Ryan TJ: Experimental angioplasty: Circumferential distribution of laser thermal energy with a laser probe. J Am Coll Cardiol 5:934–938, 1985.

15. Welch AJ, Bradley AB, Torres JH, Motamedi M, Ghidori JJ, Pearse JA, Hussein H, O'Rourke RA: Laser probe ablation of normal and atherosclerotic human aortic in vitro: A first thermographic and histologic analysis. Circulation 76:1353–1363, 1987.

16. Doubilet P, Abrams HL: The cost of underutilization. Percutaneous transluminal angioplasty for peripheral vascular disease. N Engl J Med 310:95–102, 1984.

11. Percutaneous Coronary Laser Thermal Angioplasty

Timothy A. Sanborn, M.D.

INTRODUCTION

As cardiologists, our goal in developing laser catheter delivery systems and laser techniques in experimental animals and peripheral arteries in man was to ultimately refine this technology for treatment of patients with coronary artery disease.

For the most part and as in balloon angioplasty, almost all current coronary laser catheters were developed in animal models and tested clinically in peripheral arteries before proceeding to trials in coronary arteries. However, some attempts have been made to "bypass" clinical trials in peripheral vessels and to proceed directly to feasibility studies in coronary arteries. Personally, I have found the experience in peripheral arteries to be important for demonstration of safety [1,2] and documentation of good long-term results [3] before proceeding to trials in coronary arteries. In the case of the laser-probe device, over 100 peripheral laser-assisted balloon angioplasty procedures were performed by several investigators before the first percutaneous coronary laser procedure was performed [4,5]. This peripheral experience was most helpful in the development of equipment and techniques for coronary laser procedures. Whether other laser devices will require clinical trials in peripheral arteries as extensive remains to be seen. At least for the first percutaneous coronary laser procedures, this peripheral experience was invaluable.

AIMS OF CORONARY LASER ANGIOPLASTY

As discussed in chapter 1, the two main goals of laser angioplasty are 1) to recanalize total occlusions that cannot be crossed with conventional balloon angioplasty guidewires and 2) to reduce restenosis by partially removing the obstructing lesion and/or leaving behind a smoother luminal surface.

In peripheral arteries, after initially demonstrating

feasibility, recanalization of "impossible" total occlusions with a laser device was approached first [1], as this was a goal that could be demonstrated relatively quickly and easily. Furthermore, should vessel perforation occur in these attempts, the clinical sequelae would be minimal. The second goal, reduction of restenosis, has only recently been suggested in peripheral arteries in one report [3], which was a clinical series and not a randomized clinical trial.

In the case of most percutaneous coronary laser devices, we are essentially still in the initial feasibility stages of an evaluation and there are only a few brief reports in the literature [4,5]. Some coronary laser devices, however, are now in the process of being considered for trials to test the two goals of laser angioplasty.

PERCUTANEOUS CORONARY FEASIBILITY

Although there have been a few brief reports of intraoperative laser angioplasty [6,7] the results were less than optimal because of a number of factors, including perforation and poor long-term patency due to narrow channels [6], rigid devices [7], and probably, more importantly, the lack of fluoroscopic guidance in the operating room. In addition, the real challenge of coronary laser angioplasty will be to develop the technology and techniques for percutaneous delivery of laser energy. The laser-probe device was the first to be used percutaneously in coronary arteries [4,5]; however, other devices have also now demonstrated coronary feasibility (Spears et al., unpublished results, Litvack et al., unpublished results).

Initial Laser-probe Results in Coronary Arteries

With a background in small diseased rabbit iliac arteries [8,9] and human peripheral arteries [1-3], a trial of percutaneous laser thermal angioplasty was initiated [4,5] using a miniaturized 1.7 mm diameter argon laser-heated metal cap fibroptic [Fig. 11-1) that was first tested in canine coronary arteries and post-mortem human coronary arteries. In preclinical test-

Laser Angioplasty, pages 101–110
© 1989 Alan R. Liss, Inc.

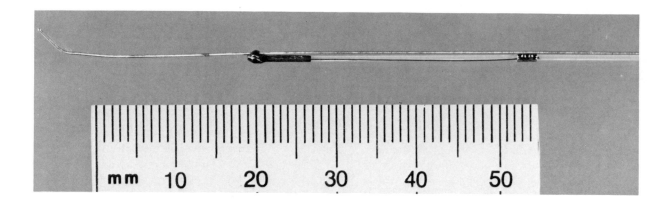

Fig. 11–1. A 1.7 mm laser-heated metal-capped fiber positioned over a 0.012 in. (0.03 cm) guidewire. A channel at the distal end of the laser probe allows it to be advanced over the guidewire. Reproduced with permission of T.A. Sanborn et al. and the American College of Cardiology (Journal of the American College of Cardiology 8:1437–1440, 1986).

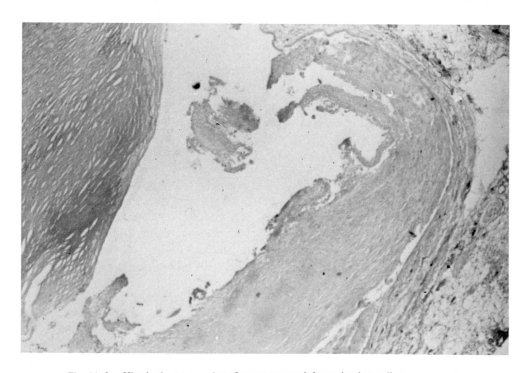

Fig. 11–2. Histologic cross section of a post-mortem left anterior descending coronary artery occlusion after recanalization with a 1.7 mm coronary laser probe using 8 W of argon laser energy for a pulse duration of 5 s. Note the lack of charring and minimal thermal damage. Hematoxylin and eosin stain. (Figure courtesy of Christian C. Haudenschild, M.D.).

ing, the device was found to have a lack of thrombogencity, spasm, or arrhythmogencity in normal canine coronary arteries. Recanalization of post-mortem occluded coronary arteries could also be accomplished without vessel perforation and surprisingly little adherence or thermal damage on histologic analysis provided the "constant-motion" technique was emphasized (Fig. 11–2).

Based on all of the above experience, clinical trials with this device were begun in Boston and Sheffield, England, with slightly different patient-selection criteria. My colleague Dr. David Cumberland took the approach of using only the laser-probe device when a coronary lesion could be crossed with a guidewire but not with a balloon catheter. With these difficult lesions, laser-assisted balloon angioplasty was accomplished in four patients using 8 W of argon laser power for 5–10 s; however, in three patients, the procedure was complicated by myocardial infarction, with two events occurring 4–12 h postprocedure. Acute thrombosis was suspected as the cause of these events.

A different approach and patient-selection criteria was chosen at Boston University. Our intent was to first demonstrate the safety and feasibility of this technique in straightforward high-grade stenosis while subjecting the patient to the least risk by keeping a guidewire distal to the stenosis for rapid balloon dilatation if necessary. The goal was only to document the safety of percutaneous coronary laser thermal angioplasty, not to prove its usefulness or effectiveness in assisting conventional balloon angioplasty. In this small series, laser-assisted balloon angioplasty was successful in four of seven patients; however, laser recanalization was unsuccessful in three stenoses because of vessel tortuosity and poor device profile with these early prototype devices. Two of these "laser failures" could be treated with more flexible balloon catheters, whereas one lesion could not be treated by any means except bypass surgery. Most importantly, no perforations, distal emboli, or myocardial infarctions occurred as a result of the additional laser procedure. Angiographic examples of two cases with these early devices are shown in Figures 11–3 and 11–4.

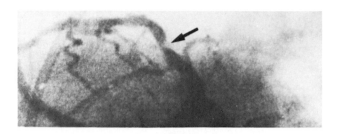

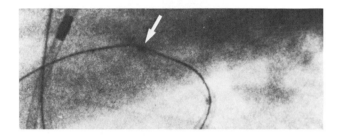

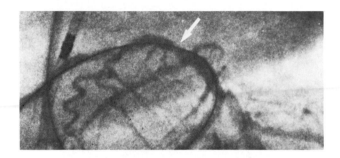

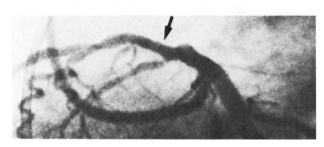

Fig. 11–3. The 60° left anterior oblique, 10° caudal views of the 90% eccentric left anterior descending coronary artery lesion (arrows) before treatment (top), after laser thermal angioplasty with the laser probe through the lesion and the angiographic result of laser thermal angioplasty (middle panels), and after balloon angioplasty (bottom). Reproduced with permission of T.A. Sanborn et al. and the American College of Cardiology (Journal of the American College of Cardiology 8:1437–1440, 1986).

Second-generation Coronary "Coil" Laser-probe Catheters

As can be appreciated from Figures 11–3 and 11–4, only lesions in straight portions of the coronary arteries were amenable to treatment with the early laser-probe devices [10]. The key catheter requirements for coronary laser angioplasty are similar to those of balloon angioplasty and include flexibility, profile, and tractability. These three factors were improved upon in the second generation of laser-probe "coil" catheters (Fig. 11–5). With improved flexibility, over 50 proximal, mid, and distal native coronary lesions as well as lesions

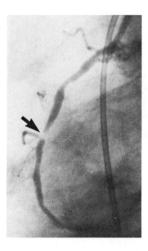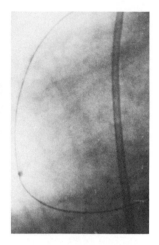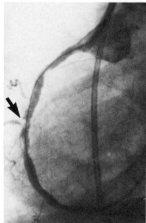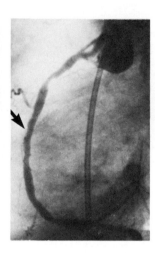

Fig. 11–4.   Angiograms of a 95% middle right coronary artery stenosis. Left panel: Before treatment. Left middle panel: Laser probe (1.7 mm) through the lesion after laser recanalization with two pulses of argon laser energy delivered for 5 s each. Right middle panel: Thirty percent residual stenosis after laser recanalization. Right panel: Ten percent residual stenosis after balloon angioplasty with a 3.0 mm balloon catheter. Flow to the acute marginal and initially interrupted after balloon angioplasty but subsequently was restored spontaneously. Reproduced with permission of T.A. Sanborn and The American Heart Association (Circulation 78:769–774, 1988).

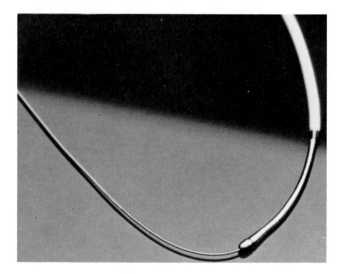

Fig. 11–5.   A 1.3 mm "flexible-coil" coronary laser probe with a central lumen containing a 0.014 in. PTCA guidewire. (Figure courtesy of Trimedyne, Inc., Santa Ana, CA.)

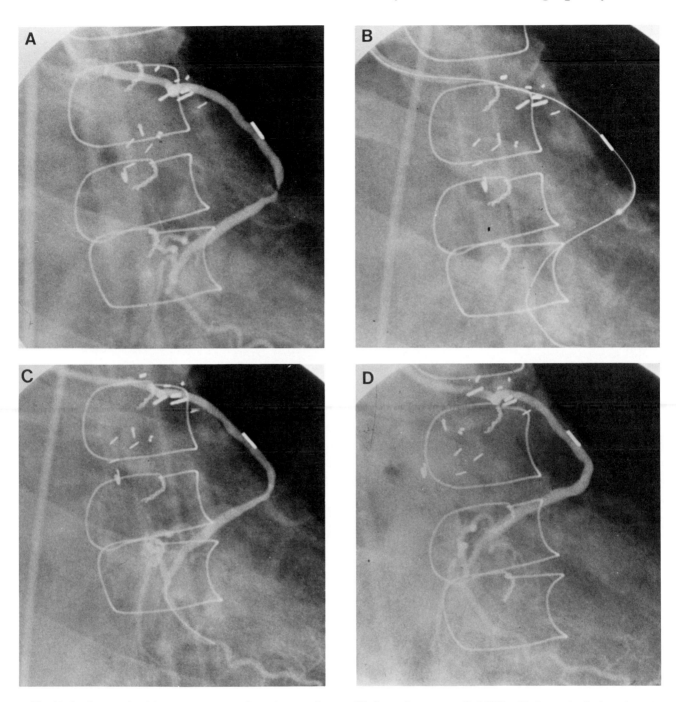

Fig. 11–6. Laser-assisted thermal angioplasty of a saphenous vein bypass graft. **A,** Ten-year-old saphenous vein bypass graft to an obtuse marginal artery with a subtotal occlusion in the body of the graft that had been dilated with conventional balloon angioplasty once before. **B,** View of the 1.6 mm laser probe across the stenosis after delivery of 12 W of argon laser energy. **C,** A 30% residual stenosis after laser thermal angioplasty with an exchange wire remaining distal to the lesion. **D,** Final result after subsequent balloon angioplasty. (Figure courtesy Dr. Thomas Linnemeier, St. Vincent's Hospital, Indianapolis, IN.)

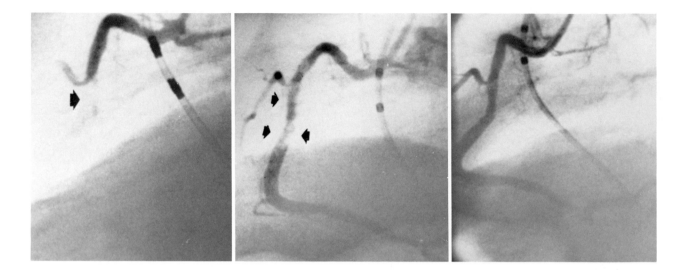

Fig. 11–7.   Example of post-PTCA laser thermal angioplasty. Left panel: A total right coronary artery occlusion in a patient with a recent inferior myocardial infarction, persistent postinfarction angina, and a partially reversible inferoapical thallium scan. Collaterals were present from the left coronary artery. Middle panel: Conventional PTCA was performed; however, residual filling defects persisted that were not re-lieved by intraarterial urokinase and 48 h of heparinization. Right panel: A 1.6 mm coronary "coil" laser probe was therefore introduced over a 0.014 in. guidewire and passed over the segment using 10 W of argon laser energy. Further balloon dilation was not required because of the excellent angiographic result with the 1.6 mm laser probe alone. (Figure courtesy of Dr. Richard Myler, San Francisco Heart Institute.)

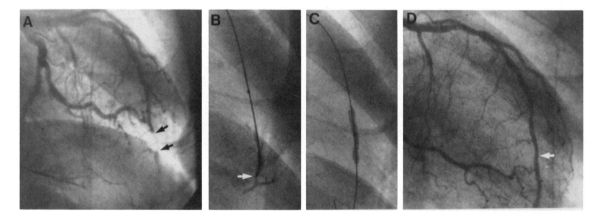

Fig. 11-8.   Recanalization of the distal LAD total occlusion which previously could not be crossed by a steerable guidewire despite balloon catheter "back up" support. **A,** The lcm occlusion (between arrows) with the distal vessel filling by bridging collaterals. **B,** Using a 0.018 inch "J" laserwire (white arrow) positioned inside a 2.0mm Sci-Med Trac Plus™ balloon catheter the occlusion was successfully recanalized with 3.0 watts of argon laser power for 3 seconds duration (9 total joules). Contrast injection through the balloon catheter confirmed that the laserwire was intraluminal (white arrow). **C,** The lesion was subsequently dilated with a 3.0mm balloon catheter. **D,** Final angiographic result with white arrow pointing to the site of the prior total occlusion. (Figures courtesy of Drs. T.A. Sanborn, J.A. Ambrose, and R. Hershman, Mount Sinai Medical Center, New York, NY.)

in saphenous vein bypasses have now been successfully treated by several investigators with minimal complications [11,12]. A few examples of cases performed by some of my colleagues are shown in Figures 11–6 and 11–7. Again, whereas these cases demonstrate feasibility, the real test of coronary laser angioplasty will be to demonstrate its usefulness in coronary total occlusions or decreasing restenosis.

The "Laserwire"

For safety reasons, all of the above cases were performed over a guidewire. If we are to try to cross total occlusions that cannot be crossed with conventional percutaneous transluminal coronary angioplasty (PTCA) equipment, then a laser device is needed that can accomplish this goal. A 0.018 in. diameter laser-

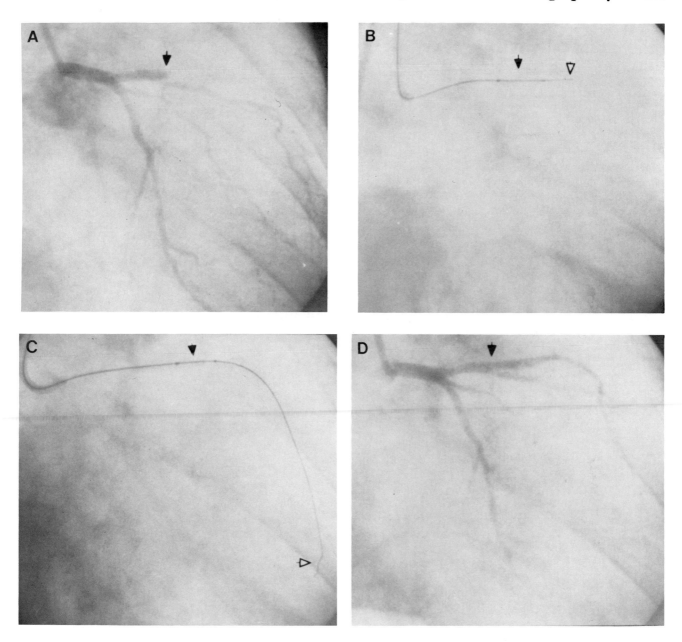

Fig. 11–9. Recanalization of a chronic total occlusion with a laser wire device. **A,** Occlusion of the left anterior descending artery in a 62-year-old man with a 4-year history of angina. No acute events or recent deterioration in symptoms was present. This occlusion could not be traversed with a flexible steerable or steerable guidewire. **B,** Using the 0.018 in. laser wire (open arrow) and 3.0 W of argon laser power, the occlusion was successfully traversed and followed by a "Profile Plus" balloon (closed arrow). **C,** A flexible steerable wire was then passed into the distal left anterior descending artery (LAD) (open arrow) so that definitive dilatation of the occlusion and a stenosis just distal to it was possible. **D,** Final angiographic result. (Figure courtesy of Drs. R. Bowes, D.C. Cumberland, and G.D.G. Oakley, Northern General Hospital, Sheffield, England.)

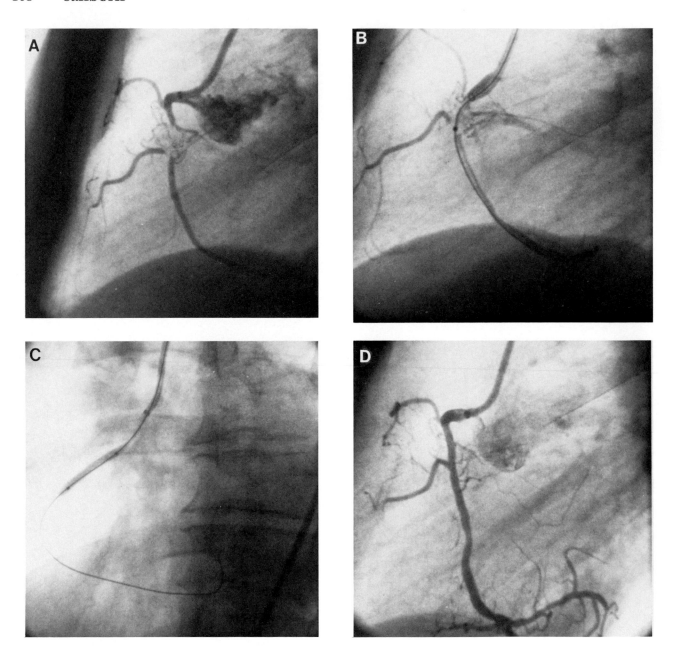

Fig. 11–10.   **A,** Example of a total right coronary artery (RCA) occlusion of at least 4 months duration recanalized with the USCI multifiber argon laser catheter. **B,** The total RCA occlusion that could be transversed with a guidewire. The laser device was therefore used over a guidewire to provide definite lumen improvement (**C**) for subsequent balloon angioplasty (**D**). (Figure courtesy of Dr. Gilles Cote, Montreal Heart Institute.)

wire that can be placed inside a balloon catheter has recently been developed and successfully used to recanalize a coronary artery total occlusion that could not be crossed with a conventional guidewire (Fig. 11–8, 11–9).

Coronary Laser-Probe Limitations and Future Directions

With these new laser-probe devices, improved initial success rates have been achieved; however, modifications of equipment and technique will undoubtedly still be required. One of the most difficult limitations that I have found, to date, is in delivering a "constant motion" to the laser probe in tortuous coronary arteries at a much greater distance from the lesion than I am accustomed to using in a superficial femoral artery occlusion only a few inches away. In order to perform this "constant-motion" technique of laser thermal angioplasty, greater axial strength and rigidity is needed in order to transmit this motion to the tip of the fiberoptic. Without this quality, the operator does not have the same one-to-one "tactile" sense and laser-probe motion is less fluid. Thus, a delicate balance between flexibility and axial rigidity must be present in a laser-probe catheter. If a device is too flexible, the operator will not be able to move the probe back and forth through a coronary lesion and adherence may occur. This has been the most difficult quality to achieve in a laser-probe catheter.

In the future, coronary laser-probe equipment and techniques will continue to be modified with different laser parameters and perhaps different catheter concepts to improve on those that exist today. Experimental studies in swine coronary arteries suggest that shorter pulse durations significantly decrease the incidence of thrombosis and platelet accumulation [13]. In fact, with 1 s laser pulses, the amount of platelet accumulation measured after use of a laser probe was no greater than that seen while advancing a conventional guidewire through the coronary artery. Additional modifications of the actual catheter should also improve the results in the future.

OTHER CORONARY LASER DEVICES

A number of other laser devices have just begun clinical trials; however, as of this writing, nothing has been published on these attempts. The various coronary laser devices currently under investigation include the Nd:YAG laser-balloon catheter used by Spears [14], the direct argon laser angioplasty systems used by Nords-trom et al. [15] and Stertzer and Cote (Fig. 11–10), and an excimer laser-system. Although all these devices are also still in the feasibility stages of development, some are being developed to address the problem of restenosis, while others are attempting to cross occlusions that cannot be treated with conventional PTCA.

CONCLUSIONS

This chapter represents a very brief but tantalizing preview of coronary laser angioplasty. It is hard to summarize the field as it is moving so rapidly. Other devices that are now being tested for feasibility in peripheral arteries include a "less thermal" excimer system [16], an Nd:YAG sapphire tip [17], a laser-induced fluorescence-guided system [18], and a rotational Nd:YAG laser system [19]. Many of these will advance to coronary trials in the near future.

REFERENCES

1. Cumberland DC, Sanborn TA, Tayler DI, Moore DJ, Welsh CL, Greenfield AJ, Guben JK, Ryan TJ: Percutaneous laser thermal angioplasty: Initial clinical results with a laserprobe in total peripheral artery occlusions. Lancet I:1457–1459, 1986.

2. Sanborn TA, Greenfield AJ, Guben JK, Menzoian JO, LoGerfo FW: Human percutaneous and intraoperative laser thermal angioplasty: Initial clinical results as an adjunct to balloon angioplasty. J Vasc Surgery 5:83–90, 1987.

3. Sanborn TA, Cumberland DC, Greenfield AJ, Welsh CL, Guben JK: Percutaneous laser thermal angioplasty: Initial results and 1-year follow-up results in 129 femoropopliteal lesions. Radiology 168:121–125, 1988.

4. Cumberland DC, Starkey IR, Oakley GDG, Fleming JS, Smith GH, Goiti JJ, Tayler DI, Davis J: Percutaneous laser-assisted coronary angioplasty. Lancet II:214, 1986.

5. Sanborn TA, Faxon DP, Kellett MA, Ryan TJ: Percutaneous coronary laser thermal angioplasty. J Am Coll Cardiol 8:1437–1440, 1986.

6. Choy DSF, Stertzer SH, Myler RK, Marco J, Forunial G: Human coronary laser recanalization. Clin Cardiol 7:377–381, 1984.

7. Livesay JJ, Leachman DR, Hagan PJ, Cooper JR, Sweeney MS, Frazier CH, Cooley DA: Preliminary report on laser coronary endarterectomy in patients (abstract). Circulation 72:III-302, 1985.

8. Sanborn TA, Faxon DP, Haudenschiuld C, Ryan TJ: Experimental angioplasty: Circumferential distribution of laser thermal energy with a laser probe. J Am Coll Cardiol 5:934–938, 1985.

110   Sanborn

9. Sanborn TA, Haudenschild CC, Faxon DP, Garber GR, Ryan TJ: Angiographic and histologic consequences of laser thermal angioplasty: Comparison with balloon angioplasty. Circulation 75:1281–1284, 1987.

10. Sanborn TA: Laser angioplasty: What has been learned from experimental studies and clinical trials? Circulation 78:769–774, 1988.

11. Sanborn TA, Bonan R, Cumberland DC, Faxon DP, Leachman DR, Linnemeier TJ, Myler RK: Percutaneous coronary laser-assisted balloon angioplasty with flexible, central lumen laserprobe catheters (abstract). Circulation 78:II–295, 1988.

12. Linnemeier TJ, Bonan R, Cumberland DC, Faxon DP, Leachman DR, Myler RK, Sanborn TA: Human percutaneous laser-assisted coronary angioplasty of saphenous vein bypass grafts: Early multicenter experience. (abstract). Circulation 78:II–295, 1988.

13. Alexopoulos D, Sanborn TA, Badimon JJ, Badimon L, Fuster V: Coronary laser thermal angioplasty: Reduced platelet accumulation, thrombi and perforations with short laser pulses (abstract). Circulation 78:II–450, 1988.

14. Spears JR: Percutaneous transluminal coronary angioplasty restenosis: Potential prevention with laser balloon angioplasty. Am J Cardiol 60:61B–64B, 1987.

15. Nordstrom LA, Castaneda-Zuniga WR, Young EG, Von Seggern, KB: Direct argon laser exposure for recanalization of peripheral arteries: Early results. Radiology 168:359–364, 1988.

16. Litvack F, Grundfest W, Mohr F, Jakubowski A, Papaioannou T, Goldenberg T, Laudenslager J, Forrester J: In vivo excimer laser angioplasty and a new, flexible blunt tipped delivery system (abstract). Circulation 76:IV-231, 1988.

17. Fourrier JL, Brunetaud JM, Prat A, Marache P, Lablanche JM, Bertrand ME: Percutaneous laser angioplasty with sapphire tip. Lancet I:105, 1987.

18. Geschwind HJ, Dubois-Rande JL, Bonner FR, Boussignac G, Prevosti LG, Leon MB: Percutaneous pulsed laser angioplasty with atheroma detection in humans (abstract). J Am Coll Cardiol 11:107A, 1988.

19. Heintzen MP, Neubaur T, Klepzig M, Zeitler E, Strauer BE: Percutaneous peripheral laser angioplasty by a novel bare fiber catheter: Initial clinical results (abstract). Circulation 76:IV-231, 1988.

12. Future Directions: Other Cardiovascular Laser Systems

Timothy A. Sanborn, M.D.

INTRODUCTION

By necessity, this volume relating the early clinical experience, equipment, and techniques in peripheral and coronary laser angioplasty has been limited essentially to a discussion of one laser delivery system as it is the only system with significant clinical experience and long-term follow-up. A few of the other laser devices are briefly mentioned at the end of the previous chapter, and although the concept of laser angioplasty is relatively new, there already is a tremendous variety of different laser approaches in various stages of experimental and clinical investigation (Table 12–1). These clinical cardiovascular laser systems are often separated by their laser wavelength (argon, Nd:YAG, CO_2, excimer, etc.); however, each laser also has the potential to be used with a variety of different delivery systems, some of which can be interchanged with other laser generators. In addition, investigators are examining a number of other approaches such as the manner in which lesions are *recognized* (angiography, angioscopy, spectroscopy, ultrasound, etc.) and the *selectivity* of atheroma for absorption of light in order to improve the effectiveness of these laser systems (Table 12–2). In the future, clinical success of the various laser angio-

plasty systems will probably depend more on the specifics of an individual fiberoptic delivery system and the pathophysiological mechanisms of action of the laser (Table 12–1). Future directions with the laser-probe systems have been alluded to in previous chapters. In this chapter, the other cardiovascular laser systems will be discussed.

ARGON LASER SYSTEMS

Another argon laser delivery system that has been developed employs a fiberoptic aligned coaxially in the center of the artery by an inflated balloon. This device also has a lens assembly at the tip of the fiberoptic to create a 40° divergent laser beam with an increased cross-sectional diameter (GV Medical, Minneapolis, MN). As in the argon laser probe clinical trials, this device is also used prior to subsequent balloon angioplasty. In an initial report [1] evaluating this device, technical success was achieved in 33 of 36 (92%) femoropopliteal and iliac stenoses and occlusions with one perforation (8%), two emboli (6%) and four abrupt reclosures (11%). Early patency at a mean of 3 months

TABLE 12–1. Characteristics and Mechanisms of Current Clinical Cardiovascular Lasers

	Lasers			
	Excimer	Argon	Nd:YAG	CO_2
Laser characteristics				
Spectral region	Ultraviolet	Visible	Near infrared	Infrared
Wavelength (nm)	308	488,514	1,060	10,600
Temporal mode	Pulsed (P)	Continuous wave (CW)	P, CW	CW
Delivery systems	Fiberoptic	Fiberoptic; metal cap; combined metal cap-sapphire tip; lensed tip	Fiberoptic; metal cap; sapphire tip; laser-balloon rotational catheter	Rigid instrument
Pathophysiological mechanisms				
Vaporization	+	+	+	+
Thermal compression	−	+	+	−
Sealing	−	−	+	−

Laser Angioplasty, pages 111–115
© 1989 Alan R. Liss, Inc.

TABLE 12–2. Current Laser Angioplasty Approaches

Modified fiberoptic tip	Improved plaque recognition
Laser probe	Angioscopy
Sapphire tip	Spectroscopy
Combined metal cap-	Ultrasound
sapphire tip	Selective plaque ablation
Lensed tip	Endogenous chromophores
Laser-balloon catheter	(carotenoids)
Short-pulse laser delivery	Exogenous chromophores
Excimer	(HPD, tetracycline)
Q-switched Nd:YAG	Other energy source
	Electrical
	Chemical

was 70%. Clinical trials in human coronary arteries have also been initiated with this device in a small number of patients.

Clinical trials with a multifiber argon laser device (USCI Division, CR Bard Inc., Billerica, MA) have also begun in human coronary arteries (see chap. 11).

Nd:YAG LASERS SYSTEMS

Experimental and Clinical Studies with Bare Nd:YAG Fiberoptics

As with the argon laser, initial in vitro and in vivo studies of Nd:YAG laser angioplasty used flexible silica fiberoptics positioned inside balloon catheters in order to maintain a central coaxial position and decrease the risk of vessel perforation [2,3]. In contrast to the previous studies with argon laser fiberoptics, a diluted blood perfusion of 3 mg/dl hemoglobin concentration was used with the Nd:YAG laser system and was found to be optimal for laser vaporization in the atherosclerotic lesion. Of note, two rapid of an infusion of saline cooled the tissue and prevented thermal injury whereas a slow rate of perfusion permitted blood to absorb the laser radiation and inhibit transfer of laser energy to the plaque.

Clinically, this Nd:YAG laser system was successful in recanalizing 12 femoropopliteal occlusions without perforation, but only narrow recanalized channels were obtained that required subsequent balloon dilation [2]. Histologic data obtained 2–4 weeks postprocedure in two patients revealed a rim of carbonization along the lumen, thermal injury, and vacuolization of the intima, and no medial or elastic tissue disruption [3].

Modified Nd:YAG Fiberoptics

Since the small (200-nm-core-diameter) fiberoptics used in the above studies created only small recanalized channels, attempts were made to modify the tips of these fiberoptics with lensed tips and sapphire contact probes in order to improve the efficacy as well as the safety of Nd:YAG laser angioplasty. In an in vitro study on human cadaver atherosclerotic arteries, a round 2.2 mm diameter sapphire contact probe was reported to be more effective than was a 1 mm diameter lensed fiberoptic [4]. In the first clinical experience with this Nd:YAG sapphire contact probe [5], successful laser recanalization to diameters of 2 mm or greater was reported in seven of eight attempts with clinical improvement in at least five patients and one laser perforation.

As this Nd:YAG laser sapphire probe represents a rounded tip that requires tissue contact for effective vaporization, it probably has a mechanism of action that is very similar to the argon laser-heated metal probe. In addition, the metal probe has recently been used and approved by the FDA for use coupled to an Nd:YAG laser. If laser recanalization with larger diameter tips of 3.5–5.0 mm is desired in order alleviate the need for subsequent balloon angioplasty, the more powerful Nd:YAG laser generator will probably be used rather than the argon laser generator. In the future, the clinical superiority of one system over the other one will depend more on various aspects of the catheter delivery system (i.e., flexibility, axial strength, and ability to pass over guidewires or "trackability").

ND:YAG Laser Sealing

An entirely different concept from the use of laser energy to recanalize occlusions prior to balloon angioplasty is the proposal [6] to apply low-level Nd:YAG laser energy after conventional balloon angioplasty to fuse or seal intimal dissections caused by balloon dilatation [7]. The rationale for this approach is twofold in that the disruptive layers of the atheroma could either collapse back into the lumen and serve as a nidus for thrombosis and *early closure* or provide the stimulus for *restenosis* through smooth muscle cell proliferation or organizing thrombus formation. In order to accomplish this goal, a fiberoptic balloon catheter was designed to transmit Nd:YAG laser radiation to a specially designed diffusing tip (USCI Division, CR Bard Inc, Billerica, MA). Laser radiation can then be dispersed radially through a relatively heat-resistant, transparent balloon catheter [6]. In vitro studies with dissected human post-mortem atheromatous iliac arteries first indicated the feasibility of this concept by demonstrating some nonuniform adherence of intima to the underlying media, and preliminary in vivo studies showed that the techniques could be applied in live animals. Whether laser sealing after balloon angioplasty can be effective clinically in preventing abrupt closure or reducing restenosis remains to be determined. Clinical trials in human coronary arteries have begun to test the feasibility of this system.

Rotational Nd:YAG Laser Catheters

As Nd:YAG laser angioplasty using bare fiberoptics is limited by the creation of only narrow channels with a high perforation rate, another laser catheter was developed with a 600 μm diameter core silica fiber fixed in an eccentric position to a central guidewire to prevent perforation [8]. In addition, by manually rotating the catheter around the guidewire during laser energy delivery, an attempt was made to create larger channels after laser angioplasty. In a preliminary report of the first clinical results with this device, peripheral laser-assisted balloon angioplasty was successful in 18 of 19 patients (14 stenoses and 5 occlusions); however, distal embolization was noted in 6 of 19 (32%) of the cases. Long-term evaluation is necessary to further evaluate this intriguing device.

CO_2 LASER SYSTEMS

Experimental Results

Historically, the CO_2 laser was shown very early to be able to vaporize atherosclerotic vessel in vitro by using a direct laser beam [9–11]. In these studies, a typical wedge-shaped laser crater similar to that produced by argon or Nd:YAG laser energy was observed. In one study [11], the long-term effects of laser irradiation on atherosclerotic tissue was performed with a CO_2 laser. In these investigations in atherosclerotic swine, the aorta was exposed through a thoracotomy and the luminal surface of the aorta rinsed for an in situ study of direct CO_2 laser irradiation. The aorta was then closed and the animals kept alive for subsequent sacrifice for histological analysis at 2 days, 2 weeks, and 8 weeks after the laser procedure. Thus, this study was the first to examine the biological response of not only the arterial wall, but also of red blood cells, leukocytes, platelets, and fibrin to laser irradiation. Two days postprocedure, the laser craters were filled with platelet-fibrin thrombi, while the healing response was characterized by reendothelization within 2 weeks and a thick fibrous cap by 8 weeks. Therefore, it was demonstrated that laser radiation could be used to ablate focal atherosclerotic lesions without inducing an excess thrombogenicity in large nonstenotic aortas.

More recently, infrared optical fibers capable of transmitting CO_2 laser energy have been developed and used both in vitro and in vivo to vaporize atherosclerotic lesions in rabbits [12]. Whether these fiberoptics can be modified so that they do not suffer the same problems of vessel perforation and small recanalized channels that have been observed with bare argon or Nd:YAG laser fiberoptics remains to be determined.

Clinical Trials

Despite the limitations and technical restrictions of a rigid device, an intraoperative coronary endarterectomy trial has begun with a hand-held CO_2 laser device, and the preliminary results have been presented [13,14]. Laser ablation of plaque was effective in relieving stenosis in 32 of 34 arterial segments for a 94% primary success rate. The laser was ineffective in two heavily calcified arteries, and surgical endarterectomy was required. Perforation occurred in two instances: one related to a balloon catheter and the other to misalignment of the laser. Both perforations could be easily repaired surgically.

On follow-up coronary angiography of these laser-treated vessels, relief of stenosis was seen in long diffuse lesions, total occlusions, and multisegmental stenosis. Early patency 1 week to 3 months postprocedure was present in 21 of 27 (78%) laser-treated arterial segments. Thrombosis occurred in the six other laser-treated arteries. Thus, intraoperative laser angioplasty with a hand-held CO_2 laser device was found to be a potential adjunct to coronary artery bypass techniques, particularly in patients with distal disease or segmental lesions. Whether this technique will represent an important intraoperative surgical technique in comparison to surgical endarterectomy and whether the success rate can be improved with more flexible fiberoptic devices remains to be determined.

Excimer Laser Systems

Experimental studies. Excimer laser radiation at the 308 nm wavelength has been used to vaporize the human cadaver atherosclerotic aorta and occluded saphenous vein bypass grafts excised at the time of repeat bypass surgery [15]. In contrast to the secondary zones of thermal and blast injury created with argon and Nd:YAG laser energy, the excimer laser-irradiated tissue had a narrow deep incision with minimal or no thermal injury. Thus, excimer lasers appear to cause tissue vaporization with less thermal damage to surrounding tissue. Whether this is a result of more precise ablation through better absorption, shorter pulse duration, sufficient time between pulses to allow tissue to cool, or a proposed photochemical rather than a photothermal laser-tissue interaction remains to be determined. Preliminary reports indicate that excimer laser recanalization can be achieved in experimentally occluded canine femoral arteries [16] and human peripheral artery occlusions (F. Litvack, personal communication). Whether decreased thermal trauma to the arterial wall will result in more or less thrombogenesis or restenosis than with thermal laser systems awaits additional experimental and clinical studies. One preliminary report indicates that surface thrombogenicity was worse with excimer as opposed to a catalytic thermal tip catheter [17].

THE CONCEPT OF SELECTIVE LASER ABLATION

All of the above lasers systems result in nonselective ablation of tissue. One additional approach to decrease vessel perforation of the arterial wall is to administer a chromaphore that is preferentially absorbed by atheroma and enhances ablation of atheroma rather than the normal arterial wall. For example, it has been shown that hematoporphyrin (HPD), which has been used in cancer photodynamic therapy, can be selectively taken up by atheroma in cholesterol-fed rabbits and that HPD activated by low-level laser radiation can cause cell necrosis in atheroma [18]. However, it remains to be determined whether HPD can be taken up in vivo by necrotic, "gruel"-type human atherosclerotic lesions. In patients undergoing vascular surgery, intravenous tetracycline administration was found to fluoresce and to enhance ultraviolet laser ablation in excised atheroma when compared to untreated tissue [19]. Whether this selective ablation or cell necrosis will be adequate to relieve obstructive lesions in vivo and not release significant embolic debris remains to be determined.

CONCLUSIONS

We are definitely entering a new era of interventional techniques. There is already evidence that at least one laser device can supplement the vascular radiologists' complement of balloons and wires to recanalizing lesions that previously could not be treated [20]. Perhaps more exciting is the suggestion that long-term results for femoropopliteal angioplasty may be improved with laser techniques [21]. We have learned that bare fiberoptics are unsafe and provide inadequate recanalized

channels. A second generation of modified fiberoptic tips offer significant improvements in safety and efficacy compared with bare fiberoptics. Pathophysiological studies have been key in determining the mechanisms of action of these devices. The improved results are attributed to self-centering rounded tips, circumferential vaporization, thermal compression by the "contact" devices, and a residual luminal surface that has less fracture, dissection, and restenosis than does balloon angioplasty. Experimental research as well as randomized comparative clinical trials are greatly needed to determine which laser devices can improve upon the two major limitations of balloon angioplasty: recanalization of chronic total occlusions and restenosis.

REFERENCES

1. Nordstrom LA, Castaneda-Zuniga WR, Young EG, Von Seggern KB: Direct argon laser exposure for recanalization of peripheral arteries: Early results. Radiology 168:359–364, 1988.
2. Geschwind HJ, Boussignac G, Teisseire B, Benhaiem N, Bittoun R, Laurent D: Conditions for effective Nd-YAG laser angioplasty. Br Heart J 52:484–489, 1984.
3. Geschwind H, Fabre M, Chaitman BR, Lefebvre-Villardebo M, Ladouch A, Boussignac G, Blair JD, Kennedy HL: Histopathology after Nd-YAG laser percutaneous transluminal angioplasty of peripheral arteries. J Am Coll Cardiol 8:1089–1095, 1986.
4. Geschwind HJ, Kern MJ, Vandormael MG, Blair JD, Deligonul U, Kennedy HL: Efficiency and safety of optically modified fiber tips for laser angioplasty. J Am Coll Cardiol 10:655–661, 1987.
5. Fourrier JL, Brunetaud JM, Prat A, Marache P, Lablanche JM, Bertrand ME: Percutaneous laser angioplasty with sapphire tip. Lancet I:105, 1987.
6. Spears JR: Percutaneous transluminal coronary angioplasty restenosis: Potential prevention with laser balloon angioplasty. Am J Cardiol 60:61B–64B, 1987.
7. Sanborn TA, Faxon DP, Haudenschild CC, Gottsman SB, Ryan TJ: The mechanism of transluminal angioplasty: Evidence for formation of aneurysm in experimental atherosclerosis. Circulation 68:1136–1140, 1983.
8. Heintzen MP, Neubaur T, Klepzig M, Zeitler E, Strauer BE: Percutaneous peripheral laser angioplasty by a novel bare fiber catheter. Initial clinical results (abstract). Circulation 76:IV-231, 1987.
9. Lee G, Ikeda RM, Kozina J, Mason DT: Laser dissolution of coronary atherosclerotic obstruction. Am Heart J 102:1074–1075, 1981.
10. Abela GS, Normann S, Cohen D, Feldman RL, Geiser EA, Conti CR: Effects of carbon dioxide, Nd:YAG, and argon laser radiation on coronary atheromatous plaque. Am J Cardiol 60:1199–1205, 1982.

11. Gerrity RG, Loop FD, Golding LAR, Ehrhart LA, Argenyi ZB: Arterial response to laser operation for removal of atherosclerotic plaques. J Thorac Cardiovasc Surg 85:409–421, 1983.

12. Eldar M, Battler A, Neufeld HN, Gaton E, Arieli R, Akselrod S, Levite A, Katzir A: Transluminal carbon dioxide-laser catheter angioplasty for dissolution of atherosclerotic plaques. J Am Coll Cardiol 3:135–137, 1984.

13. Livesay JJ, Leachman DR, Hagan PJ, Cooper JR, Sweeney MS, Frazier CH, Colley DA: Preliminary report on laser coronary endarterectomy in patients (abstract). Circulation 72:III-302, 1985.

14. Livesay JJ: Laser coronary angioplasty. Cardiac Chron 1:1–4, 1986.

15. Grundfest WS, Litvack F, Goldenberg T, Sherman T, Morenstern L, Carroll R, Fisbein M, Forrester J, Margitan J, McDermid S, Pacala TJ, Rider DM, Laudenslager JB: Pulsed ultraviolet laser and the potential for safe laser angioplasty. Am J Surg 150:220–226, 1985.

16. Forrester JS, Litvack F, Grundfest WS: Laser angioplasty and cardiovascular disease. Am J Cardiol 57:990–992, 1986.

17. Prevosti LG, Lawrence JB, Leon MB, Smith PD, Lu DY, Kramer WS, Clark RE: Surface thrombogenicity after excimer laser and hot-tip thermal ablation of plaque: Morphometric studies using an anular perfusion chamber. Surg Forum 33:330–333, 1987.

18. Litvack F, Grundfest WS, Forrester JS, Fishbein MC, Swan HJC, Corday E, Rider DM, McDermid IS, Pacala TH, Laudenslager JB: Effects of hematoporphyrin derivative and photodynamic therapy on atherosclerotic rabbits. Am J Cardiol 56:667–671, 1985.

19. Murphy-Chutorian D, Kosek J, Mok W, Quay S, Huestis W, Mehigan J, Profitt D, Ginsburg R: Selective absorption of ultraviolet laser energy by human atherosclerotic plaque treated with tetracycline. Am J Cardiol 55:1293–1297, 1985.

20. Cumberland DC, Sanborn TA, Taylor DI, Moore DJ, Welsh CL, Greenfield AJ, Guben JK, Ryan TJ: Percutaneous laser thermal angioplasty: Initial clinical results with a laserprobe in total peripheral artery occlusions. Lancet I:1457–1459, 1986.

21. Sanborn TA, Cumberland DC, Welsh CL, Greenfield AJ, Guben JK: Percutenaous laser thermal angioplasty: Initial results and one year follow-up results in 129 femoropoliteal lesions. Radiology 168:121–125, 1988.

INDEX

★ IT'S MY STATE! ★
New Hampshire

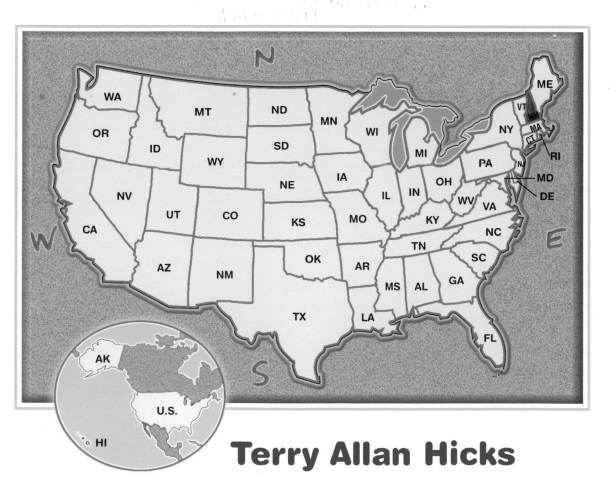

Terry Allan Hicks

BENCHMARK BOOKS

MARSHALL CAVENDISH
NEW YORK

To Dr. and Mrs. George Brown, my first (and still my favorite) New Hampshirites

Benchmark Books
Marshall Cavendish
99 White Plains Road
Tarrytown, New York 10591-9001
www.marshallcavendish.com

Library of Congress Cataloging-in-Publication Data

Hicks, Terry Allan.
New Hampshire / by Terry Allan Hicks.
p. cm. — (It's my state!)
Includes bibliographical references and index.
ISBN 0-7614-1825-3
1. New Hampshire—Juvenile literature. I. Title. II. Series.

F34.3.H53 2004
974.2—dc22
2004010634

Photo research by Candlepants Incorporated

Front Cover: Mike Brinson / The Image Bank / Getty Images
Back cover illustration: The license plate shows New Hampshire's postal abbreviation, followed by its year of statehood.

The photographs in this book are used by permission and through the courtesy of: *Corbis:* 34, 35; James Randklev, 4 (top), 70; Eric and David Hosking, 4 (bottom); Wolfgang Kaehler, 5 (top); Robert Pickett, 5 (bottom); Lee Snider, 9, 50, 57, 66; Steve Terrill, 12; Bob Krist, 13, 52; Christopher J. Morris, 17; David Muench, 18; Phil Schermeister, 19, 51; W. Perry Conway, 20 (top); D. Robert & Lorri Franz, 20 (middle); Joe McDonald, 21 (middle); Peter Blakely, 40; Brooks Kraft, 41 (bottom); Kevin Fleming, 42, 46; Fotografia, Inc., 44; Rick Friedman, 45, 59; Dan Habib / Concord Monitor, 47; Sygma, 48 (bottom); E.O. Hoppe, 49 (top); Erik Freeland, 53; Dave G. Houser, 64; Mark Peterson, 65; Bettmann, 33, 49 (middle), 49 (bottom). *Photo Researchers, Inc.:* Jim Zipp, 4 (middle); Mark A. Schneider, 5 (middle); Scott-Berthoule, 22; Larry West, 23. *Index Stock:* Bill Bachmann, 8; Steve Dunwell, 10; Glenn Kulbako, 11; Kindra Clineff, 14; David White, 15; Paul Johnson, 16; Frank Siteman, 60; Greig Cranna, 63, 68 (top); Steven Saks, 71; John Coletti, 72. *Minden Pictures:* Jim Brandenburg, 20 (bottom); Tim Fitzharris, 21 (top). *Animals Animals / Earth Scenes:* Michael S. Bisceglie, 21 (bottom). *The Image Works:* Julie Henderson, 48 (top); Joe Sohm, 54. *Getty Images:* Digital Vision, 68 (middle); Lester Lefkowitz / Taxi, 68 (bottom); Photodisc Blue, 69 (top). *Envison:* Photononstop, 69 (middle); Steven Needham, 69 (bottom). *North Wind Picture Archives:* 30, 31, 32, 41 (top). *Special Collections Department, Bailey Howe Library, University of Vermont:* 24. *Lewis Hine Collection / Photography Collection Albin O. Kuhn Library / University of Maryland, Baltimore County:* 36. *New Hampshire Historical Society:* 28, 48 (middle). *Portsmouth Naval Shipyard Museum:* 38.

Book design by Anahid Hamparian

Printed in Italy

1   3   5   6   4   2

Contents

A Quick Look at New Hampshire

Nickname: The Granite State
Population: 1,288,000 (2003 estimate)
Statehood: June 21, 1788

Tree: White Birch

This tall, graceful tree is sometimes called the canoe birch, because the Native Americans made fast, lightweight canoes from its bark. Because real paper was expensive and hard to find, New Hampshire's early settlers sometimes wrote on birch bark.

Bird: Purple Finch

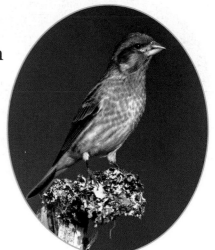

This brightly colored bird is a favorite of many of the state's farmers and gardeners. Purple finches eat many insects that can harm plants and crops. The purple finch has been the state's official bird since 1957.

Flower: Purple Lilac

Benning Wentworth, the first colonial governor of New Hampshire, planted these showy flowers, which were imported from England, at his house in 1750. The lilac's big, sweet-smelling blossoms are now one of the most welcome signs of spring in New Hampshire.

4

Animal: White-Tailed Deer

New Hampshire's state animal is named for its white-edged tail. The deer raises its tail when it feels threatened to alert other deer to danger. Some experts estimate that more than 70,000 white-tailed deer live in the state today.

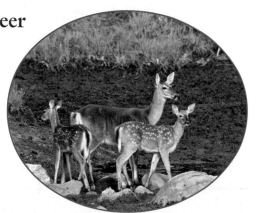

Rock: Granite

Granite quarrying (taking granite from the ground) was once an important New Hampshire industry. The Washington Monument, parts of New York's Brooklyn Bridge, and the cornerstone of the United Nations Building are all made of New Hampshire granite.

Insect: Ladybug

In 1975, the fifth-grade students at Broken Ground School in Concord started a petition for their choice of state insect, the ladybug. Two years later, the state legislature chose the ladybug.

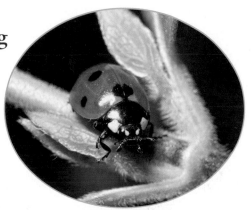

NEW HAMPSHIRE

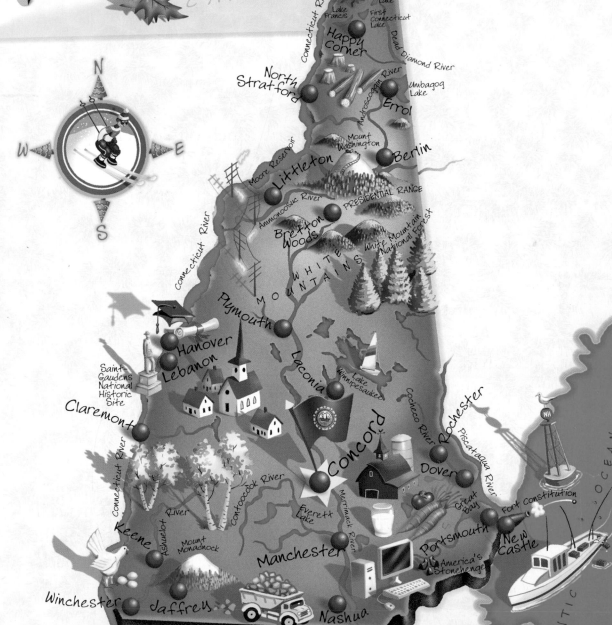

CANADA

N W E S

Second Connecticut Lake

Lake Francis

First Connecticut Lake

Connecticut River

Happy Corner

Dead Diamond River

North Stratford

Androscoggin River

Umbagog Lake

Errol

Mount Washington

Berlin

Moore Reservoir

Littleton

Ammonoosuc River

PRESIDENTIAL RANGE

Bretton Woods

White Mountain National Forest

WHITE MOUNTAINS

Connecticut River

Plymouth

Laconia

Lake Winnipesaukee

Rochester

Hanover

Cocheco River

Lebanon

Piscataqua River

Saint-Gaudens National Historic Site

OCEAN

Claremont

Concord

Dover

Connecticut River

Merrimack River

Great Bay

Fort Constitution

Ashuelot River

Everett Lake

Contoocook River

Portsmouth

New Castle

Keene

Mount Monadnock

Manchester

America's Stonehenge

ATLANTIC

Winchester

Jaffrey

Nashua

1 The Granite State

With an area of just 9,304 square miles, New Hampshire is the fourth-smallest state in the country. Much of New Hampshire's landscape was formed thousands of years ago by retreating glaciers (large slow-moving masses of ice) and a harsh climate. Over time, wind and water helped to shape the state. New Hampshire can be divided into three main regions: the Coastal Lowlands, the Eastern New England Upland, and the White Mountains.

New Hampshire's Borders
North: Canada
South: Massachusetts
East: Maine
West: Vermont and Canada

The Coastal Lowlands

New Hampshire has barely eighteen miles of seacoast, where the Piscataqua River meets the Atlantic Ocean. It was here, in the Coastal Lowlands, that Europeans first settled. One of the towns they built, Strawbery Banke (now called Portsmouth) grew into one of America's great shipbuilding centers and New Hampshire's first capital.

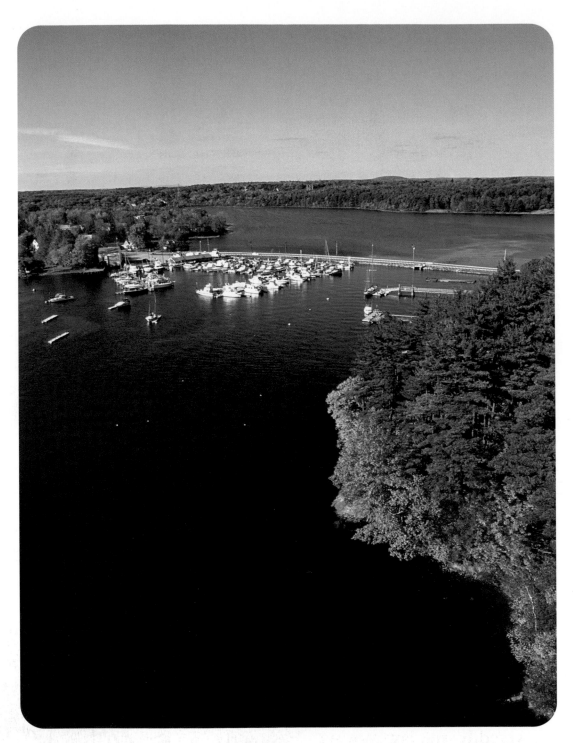

The mouth of the Piscataqua River, at Portsmouth, has welcomed ships for centuries. It is still a popular place for pleasure boating and fishing.

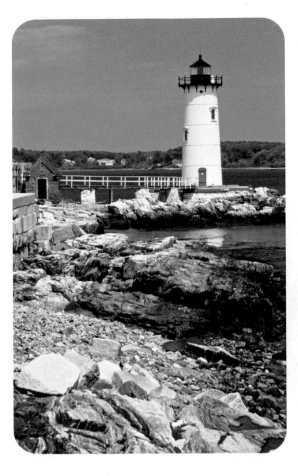

The Portsmouth Harbor Lighthouse has stood on New Castle, at the mouth of the Piscataqua River, since 1771.

Portsmouth is still a working seaport, and the seacoast is now an important tourist destination. One of the best-known attractions of this region is the Isles of Shoals, six miles out in Piscataqua Bay. These beautiful islands feature a famous garden created by the nineteenth-century poet Celia Thaxter, as well as a marine research laboratory that studies the life in the surrounding waters.

The Eastern New England Upland

About half of New Hampshire is taken up by the Eastern New England Upland. Most of the state's major cities and towns—including Manchester, Nashua, and the state capital, Concord—are found in the river valleys of the Upland. In the early 1900s, factories and mills began to appear here, powered by the fast-moving Merrimack River.

New Hampshire is sometimes called "the Mother of Rivers," because five of New England's great rivers—the Androscoggin, Connecticut, Merrimack, Piscataqua, and Saco—begin here. In all, the state has more than 40,000 miles of rivers.

Most of the state's once-famous granite quarries are found in the Upland, especially around Concord. This area also has many fruit and dairy farms. New Hampshire has around 1,300 lakes or ponds. The Upland is home to the largest of these lakes. This includes Lake Winnipesaukee, the state's biggest lake. The lake stretches almost 80 square miles and draws thousands of tourists, especially in the summertime.

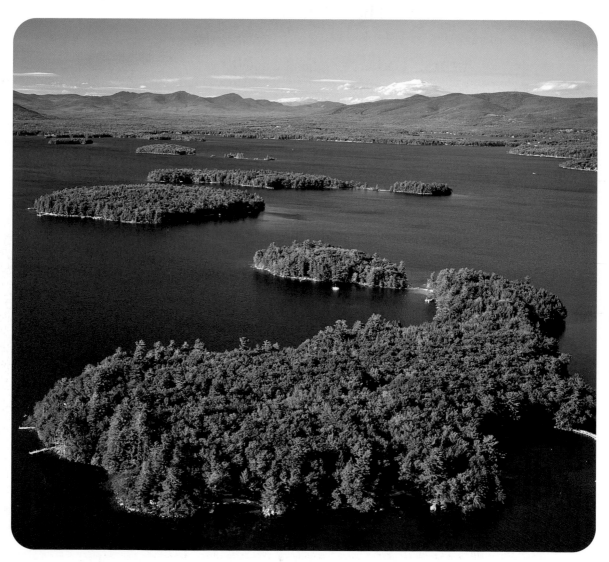

Lake Winnipesaukee is New Hampshire's largest body of water.

The strangest sights in the New Hampshire landscape might be the monadnocks. These tall, isolated hills made of rock were too hard to be worn down by the moving glaciers. The highest,

The town of Salem is home to Mystery Hill, which is also known as "America's Stonehenge." This complicated maze of stone walls and chambers—which could have been used as a solar calendar to mark the passing seasons—may be around four thousand years old. But who built it? Nobody knows for sure.

Mount Monadnock, has been a favorite of hikers since the nineteenth century. Today, about 125,000 people make the 3,165-foot climb to its peak every year.

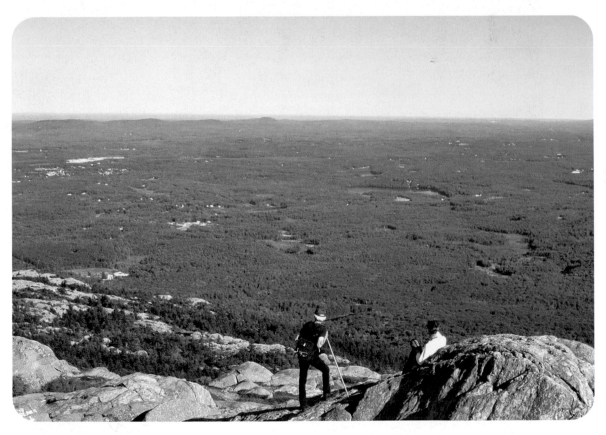

Hikers who make it to the higher areas of Mount Monadnock are treated to a spectacular view

The White Mountains

The White Mountains are named for their chalk peaks, which shine a brilliant white, even in the summertime. They take up the northern third of New Hampshire. The dense forests that cover the mountainsides supply lumber for construction and wood pulp for paper. The steep mountain valleys in this region are called notches. Tourists come here year-round. In the summer, the mountains are ideal for hiking and whitewater kayaking. In the winter, deep, powdery snow welcomes skiers.

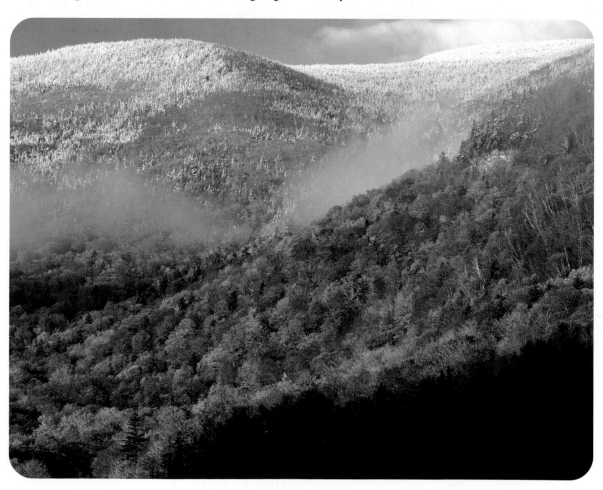

Early-morning mist covers Kinsman Mountain, part of the White Mountains. The Appalachian Trail crosses its 4,363-foot peak.

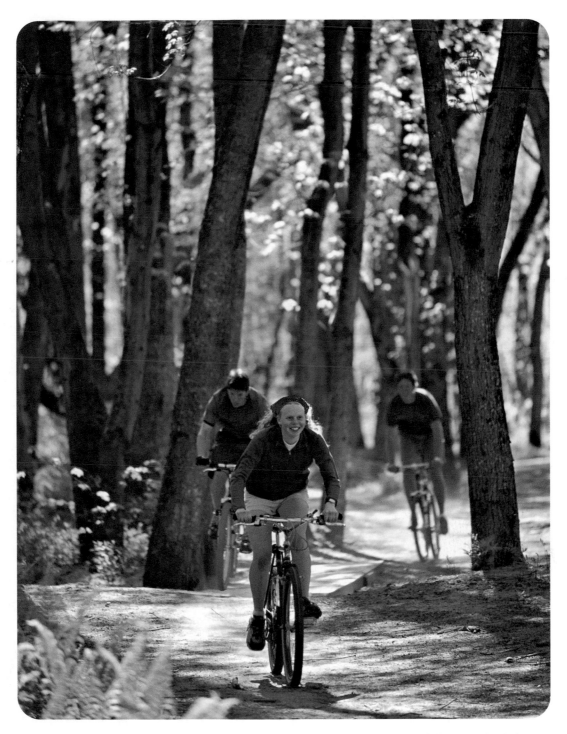

Many New Hampshirites and visitors enjoy riding mountain bikes on the bike trails in the state's forests.

The best-known section of the White Mountains is the Presidential Range, which has six peaks. All of the peaks are named for former presidents, and each is more than one mile high. One of the peaks, the 6,288-foot Mount Washington, is the tallest mountain in the northeastern United States. Visitors come here in the warm weather to ride the little steam-powered trains of the Mount Washington Cog Railway. Trains have been chugging up and down the steep mountainside since 1869.

But it was farther north, in the Franconia Range, where nature created New Hampshire's most beloved symbol: the world-famous Old Man of the Mountain. This rock formation was carved into the side of Profile Mountain near Franconia Notch by centuries of wind and rain. It looked exactly like the face of a proud, tough old man.

Imagine how shocked the people of New Hampshire were on May 3, 2003, when they discovered that the Old Man of the Mountain was gone. The rocks that made up the famous face had fallen to the valley below, perhaps worn down by years of wind, rain, and snow. The state government is now trying to decide whether this natural formation can be rebuilt—or whether anyone should even try.

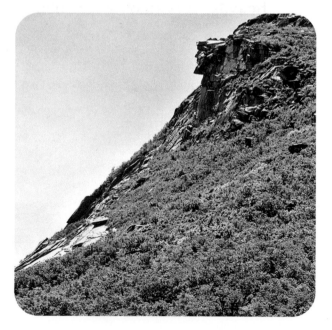

From a distance, the jutting rocks resembled an old man's face.

The Climate

New Hampshire's weather is not for everyone. The state is delightful in the spring, when the purple lilacs are in bloom and the many apple and cherry trees are covered with blossoms. The spring is usually the rainiest season for the state. New Hampshire receives about 45 inches of rain in an average year, with much higher amounts in the White Mountains.

The weather is usually cool and pleasant in the summertime, too. The average temperature during the summer is about 70 degrees Fahrenheit. The highest temperature ever recorded in NH—in 1911— was 106 degrees.

For many people, New Hampshire is at its best in the fall, when the trees of this heavily wooded state blaze with brilliant red, gold, and yellow leaves. The average high temperature in October is 60 degrees. But at night, the temperature drops to an average of 34 degrees — just above freezing.

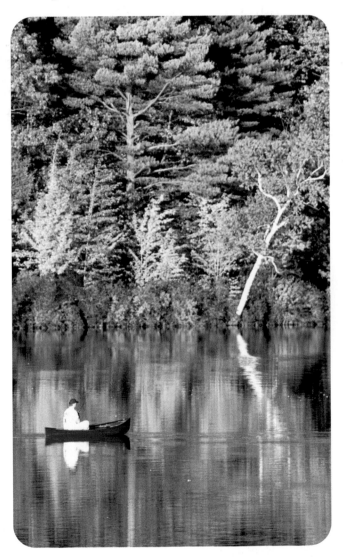

Many New Hampshirites enjoy fishing on a quiet lake in autumn.

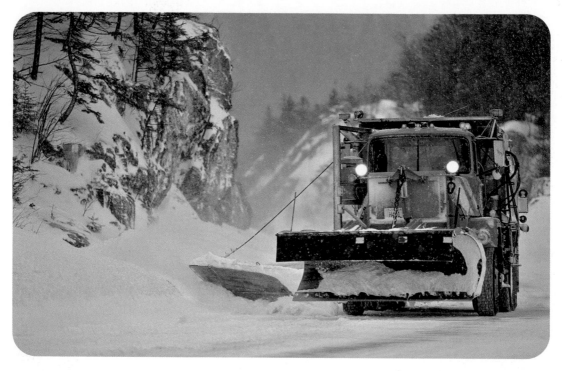

New Hampshirites are used to driving in tough winter weather. When a big storm comes, snowplows work to keep the roads clear.

The winters are another story. In midwinter, the temperature in the northern part of the state averages a bone-chilling 16 degrees Fahrenheit. There is plenty of snow, too, with an average snowfall in the northern mountains of more than 100 inches a year. The people of the state have learned to adapt to their long, cold winters. Even so, says Pattilee Leavitt, who grew up in the town of Rochester, "The best thing about a New Hampshire winter is the way is makes you appreciate a New Hampshire spring."

Mount Washington has been described as having "the most treacherous climate in the world." The weather observatory at the top of the mountain has seen some amazing weather conditions, including the highest wind ever recorded: 231 miles per hour, on April 12, 1934.

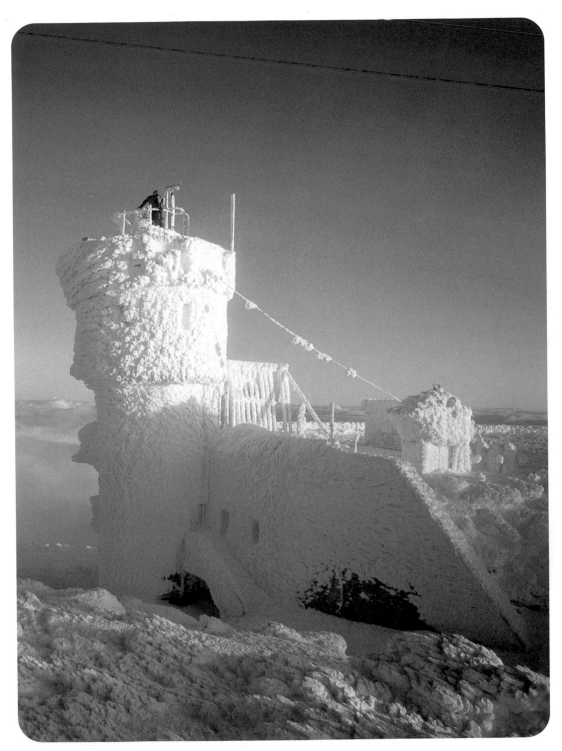

Snow and ice cover a weather station at the Mount Washington Observatory.

The Granite State

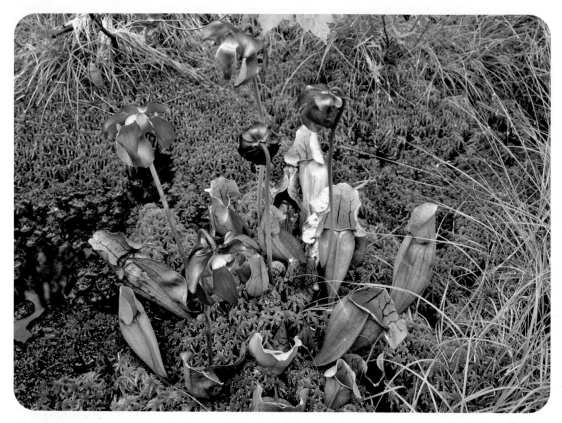

Pitcher plants can live in the swampy areas near the White Mountains.

Life in the Wild

New Hampshire is home to a dazzling variety of wildlife, both plants and animals. More than 84 percent of the state is covered by forests. The trees in the northern part of New Hampshire are mostly evergreens, such as fir and spruce. In the central and southern parts of the state, the forests are mixed, with white pine, maple, oak, and the New Hampshire state tree: the white birch.

When spring comes, hundreds of different species of wildflowers begin to appear, including trillium, pink lady's slippers, asters, buttercups, and blue, yellow, and white violets. Wild shrubs, such as mountain laurel and blueberry bushes, grow here, too.

New Hampshire

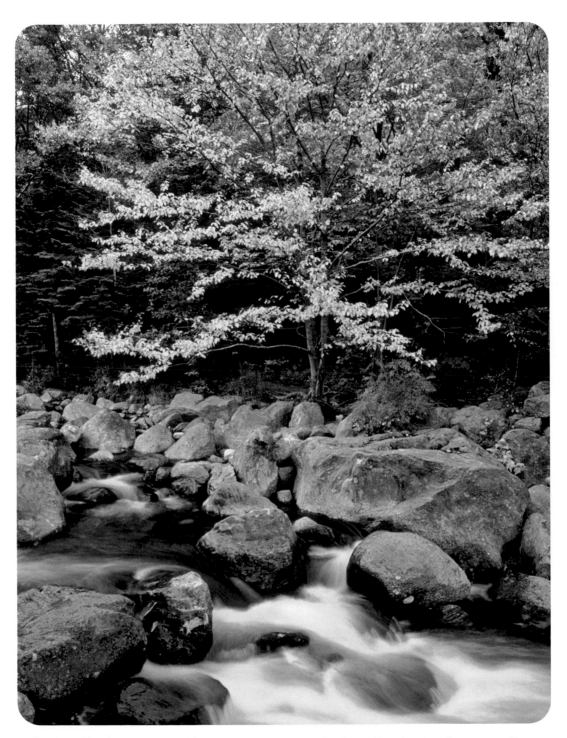

New Hampshire's deep green forests and cool, clear streams are home to all kinds of wildlife.

The Granite State

Plants & Animals

Beaver

This hardworking, highly intelligent animal builds huge mounds and dams that block rivers and ponds. Beavers were hunted almost to extinction in New Hampshire. But in recent years their numbers in the state have started to rise.

Bald eagle

In 1989, when a nesting pair of bald eagles was spotted on the shores of Lake Umbagog, it was big news all over New Hampshire. This is because these magnificent birds of prey had not been seen nesting in the state for forty years. They are still on the endangered species list, but many people are hoping there will be more of them in the future.

Black bear

The black bear is a shy creature that prefers deep woods with few humans nearby, so New Hampshire's forests make the perfect habitat for it. A black bear may weigh as much as 250 pounds. Some experts estimate that there are almost five thousand of these huge mammals in the state.

Fisher

Fishers are sometimes called "fisher-cats" in New Hampshire, even though they do not catch fish and they are not cats. The fisher's thick, glossy fur was highly prized by trappers, so the fisher population decreased. Recently, however, their population has started to increase.

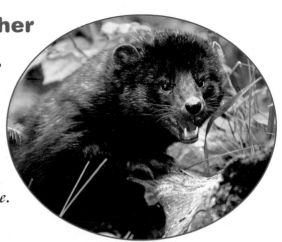

Pink Lady's Slipper

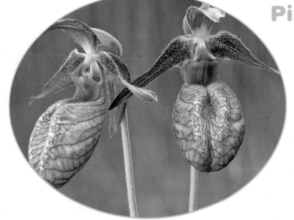

This delicate wild orchid—New Hampshire's official wildflower since 1991—is sometimes called the moccasin flower. Its leaves fold over to hide a single blossom that looks like a little shoe.

Lupine

The wild lupine can be found almost everywhere in the state, but its habitat is shrinking as the human population grows. New Hampshire's official butterfly, the Karner blue, depends on the wild lupine as food for its survival.

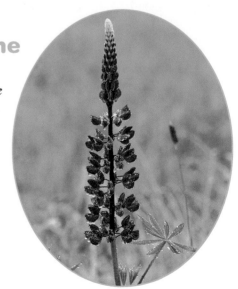

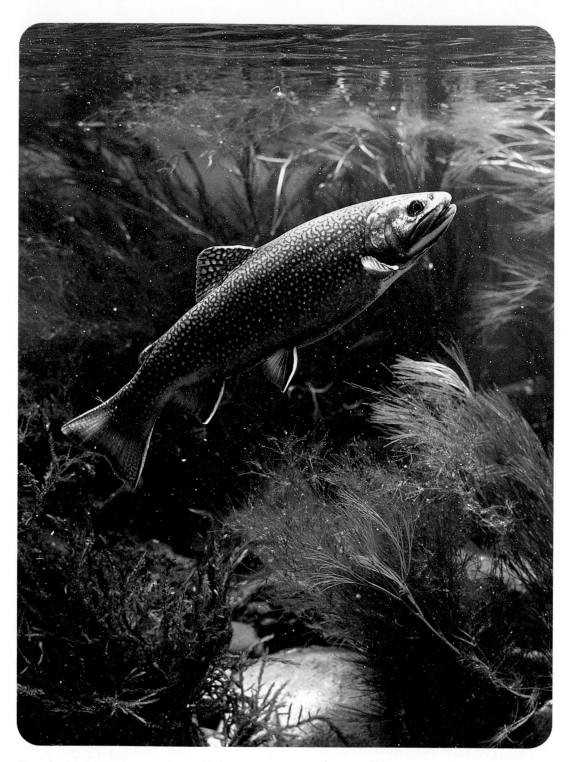

Brook trout are a popular catch for New Hampshire fishermen.

New Hampshire

Black bears, white-tailed deer, elk, and moose can be found all over the state, as well as such less-common animals as the marten and the Canadian lynx. Many game birds, such as grouse, wild turkey, and woodcock, also make their homes in New Hampshire.

The mountain ponds of northern New Hampshire are filled with brook trout. The lakes in the center of the state have many other species of trout, as well as certain types of salmon and small-mouth bass. The waters off the seacoast are also rich with life. Fish such as striped bass and bluefish live in these waters. Marine mammals such as dolphins, porpoises, and sometimes even whales also live in the coastal waters.

Unfortunately, the news for wildlife in New Hampshire is not all good. The state takes good care of its wildlife, but the spreading human habitation and pollution—especially air pollution, from other states and from Canada—are threats to New Hampshire's wildlife. A number of species, including the Canada lynx, and the timber rattlesnake, are endangered. The Karner blue butterfly and the state's Sunapee trout are also on the endangered species list. But scientists and concerned residents continue to work toward finding ways to protect the state and its wildlife.

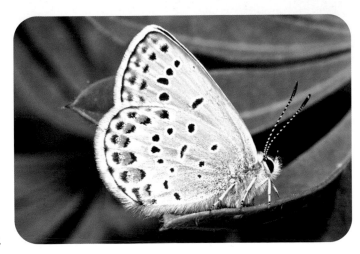

The Karner blue butterfly is New Hampshire's state insect.

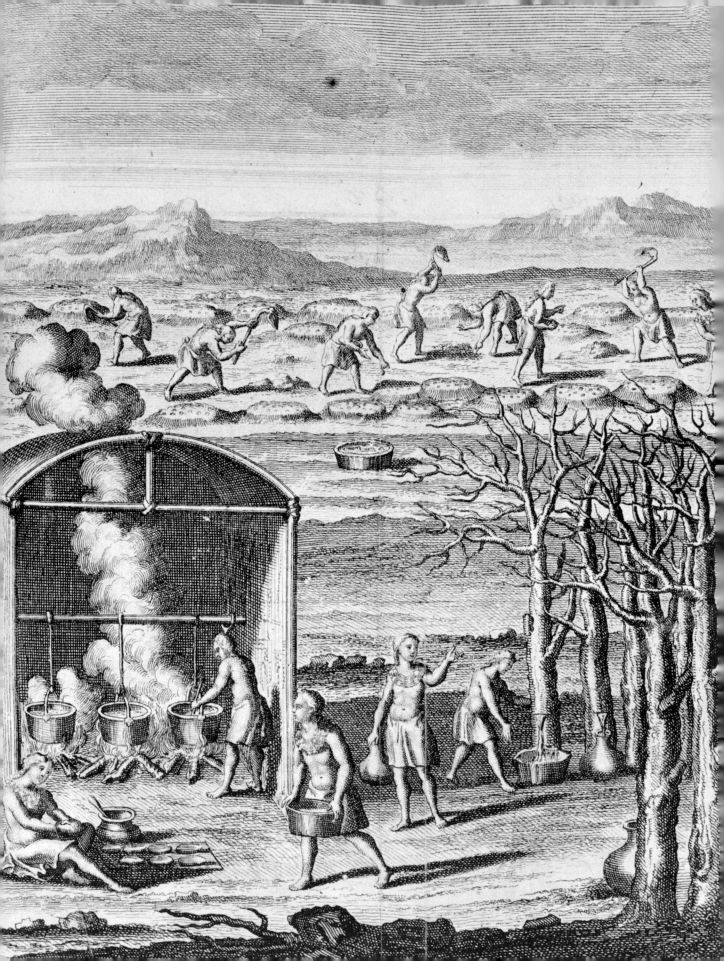

2 From the Beginning

The First People

People have been living in what is now New Hampshire since the glaciers melted away, more than ten thousand years ago. Archeologists have found Native American weapons and tools near Lake Winnipesaukee that date back as far as 7000 B.C.E.

By the early seventeenth century C.E., when Europeans first arrived, the New Hampshire area was home to about five thousand Native Americans. These people farmed, fished, and hunted wild game such as deer. Most of these Native Americans belonged to the Western Abenaki nation, which was an Algonquian-speaking group of Native Americans. The New Hampshire Native American groups, the Piscataqua, Nashua, Pennacook, Coosuc, and Ossipee, usually lived in peace with one another. They did, however, sometimes go to war against their traditional enemies. These enemies included the Iroquois, who lived to the north and west of them.

The Abenaki grew crops on their land and tapped the maple trees for syrup.

Make a Model Birch Bark Canoe

The white bark of the birch tree was an important material for many Native Americans who lived in the northeastern part of what is now the United States. From this bark they made canoes, wigwams, and baskets.

You Will Need
A large piece of heavy watercolor paper
White toilet paper
A black colored pencil
A paintbrush
Water
About 3 feet of twine, raffia, or long, dried grass or reeds
A hole puncher
A pen

To make the birch bark paper:

Use the colored pencil to draw wavy black lines and dots on the watercolor paper. Paint the entire sheet of watercolor paper with water. Lay strips of toilet paper on top of the wet watercolor paper. (The water will make the tissue crinkle to resemble peeling birch bark.) Set the paper aside to dry. Once it is dry, the toilet paper will stick to the watercolor paper.

To make the model canoe:

Fold the watercolor paper in half and cut out a pattern of the canoe in the shape of the diagram on the next page. (You can make the pattern as large or as small as you like.)

Pile the two cutouts on top of each other so that the edges line up exactly. Using the hole puncher, punch holes along the bottom and sides of both of the cutouts.

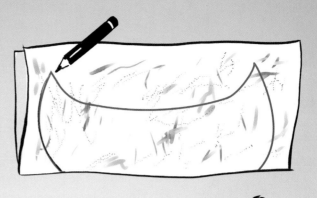

Lace the twine through the holes so that the two halves of the canoe are tied together. At each end make a knot and cut off the extra twine. Separate and spread out the two pieces top of the canoe.

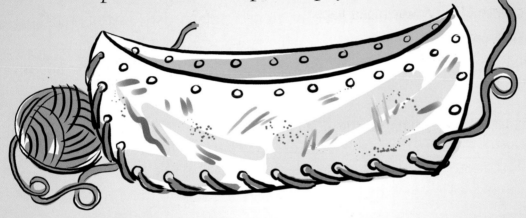

Use the ball point pen to poke small holes along the upper edges of the canoe (on both pieces.) Lace small pieces of twine in and out of the holes on one side. Do the same to the other side and do not lace the two halves together. When you are finished you can show your family and friends your canoe and imagine what it was like to paddle through New Hampshire's rivers and lakes.

The Europeans

The first non-Native American visitors to the area were probably Vikings. These sailors from Scandinavia (a part of northern Europe) began exploring the Atlantic Coast around the tenth century. Strange markings on a rock near the town of Hampton may be runes (Viking writing) that were carved around 1100 C.E.

Early European explorers, including Giovanni da Verrazano and Samuel de Champlain, sailed along the New Hampshire seacoast. But it was the English sea captain John Smith who first brought the area to the world's attention. In 1614, he visited the Isles of Shoals and the nearby seacoast. Later, he wrote that the English should settle there, saying, ". . . here every man may be master and owner of his labor and land in a short time . . ."

In 1622, the English king gave a huge piece of land in New England to Captain John Mason and Sir Ferdinando Gorges. In 1629, the two men divided up the land. Mason took the section between the Merrimack and Piscataqua rivers and named it New Hampshire, after his home county of Hampshire in England. Gorges's section eventually became the state of Maine.

Settlers began arriving in the area at the mouth of the Piscataqua in the early 1620s. A small group built Pannaway Plantation, at Odiorne's Point,

Mason and Gorges divide the land that would become New Hampshire and Maine.

near the present-day town of Rye. Around 1630, another group settled at a place they called Strawbery Banke. The settlement was named for the wild berries that grew there. Years later, the town would be known as Portsmouth.

These settlers came in search of fish to catch, land to farm, and trees to cut. They built salt works for preserving fish, and saw mills to cut lumber for houses and ships. In the early years, they usually got along well with the Native Americans. But by the 1670s, as more and more of their land was being taken by settlers, the Native Americans realized their way of life was threatened and the time of peace came to an end.

War and Revolution

Beginning in the late seventeenth century, England fought a long, bloody war with its great rival, France, for control of North America. Many Native American groups took the side of the French in this conflict, which came to be known as the French and Indian Wars.

The first major attack of the French and Indian Wars came in New Hampshire, in 1689. A group of Native American warriors— angry because hundreds of their people had been captured and sold into slavery—killed twenty-three settlers in the town of Dover. Many New Hampshire soldiers fought in the wars that followed, including five hundred men who helped capture the French fortress at Louisbourg, in present-day Nova Scotia, in 1758. The French and Indian Wars finally came to

The French and Indian Wars were a disaster for the Native Americans of New Hampshire. Many were killed in the fighting, and many more fled to Canada. By the end of the eighteenth century, most of New Hampshire's Native Americans were gone.

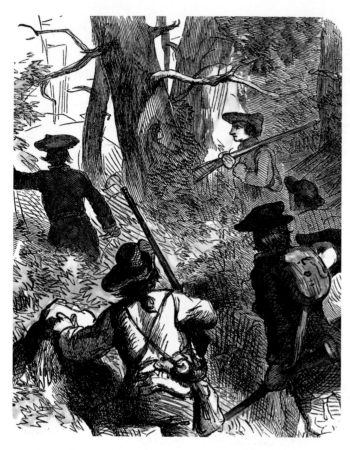

Colonial militia cross the mountains during the French and Indian War.

an end in 1763, when the French signed the Treaty of Paris, giving their colonies in Canada to the British. Peace returned to New Hampshire, but it did not last long.

The people of the colonies had been unhappy with their rulers in Britain for a long time. In the 1770s, their anger at unfair government and high taxes—some of which were meant to pay the cost of the French and Indian Wars—led to the Revolutionary War.

The first attack against the British government came in New Hampshire. On December 14, 1774, four hundred men took over Fort William and Mary, on the island of New Castle. They captured weapons and one hundred barrels of "the king's gunpowder"—some of which was probably used against the British six months later, at the Battle of Bunker Hill.

In 1769, Dartmouth College, now one of the oldest universities in the United States, opened its doors. Eleazar Wheelock, a minister, founded Dartmouth as a school for young Native Americans. In the years since, Dartmouth, in Hanover, has become one of the most respected institutions of higher learning in the country.

Then, in January 1776, New Hampshire became the first of the colonies to write its own constitution and form an independent government. Many New Hampshire men—about five thousand in all—fought in the Revolution.

One of America's finest military leaders during the Revolution was John Stark. Stark led the American forces to victory at the Battle of Bennington in Vermont, early in the war. Many years later, as an old man, he wrote a letter containing the words that would become New Hampshire's motto: "Live free or die."

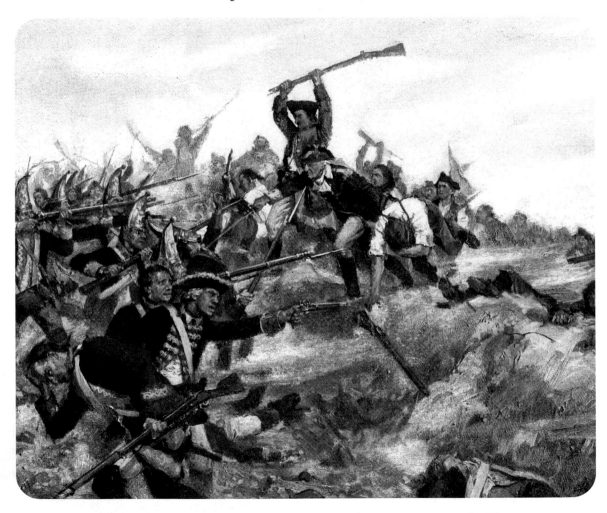

Many New Hampshirites fought bravely at the Battle of Bennington in Vermont.

When the Revolutionary War ended, New Hampshire was still at the forefront of change. On June 21, 1788, New Hampshire cast the ninth vote in favor of the Constitution. This was the deciding vote that ensured that this list of rights and rules would become law. New Hampshire was the ninth state to join the new country.

The Revolutionary War was followed by more than fifty years of peace and prosperity in New Hampshire. But in the middle of the nineteenth century, the conflict that divided the entire country—the struggle over slavery—took a terrible toll on the Granite State.

The town of Portsmouth, New Hampshire's first capital, played an important role in the Revolution. Portsmouth's shipyards built warships for the American navy. One of these was the *Ranger,* which John Paul Jones sailed all the way across the ocean to make a daring attack on Britain itself. But many people in Portsmouth sided with the British. This was one of the reasons the state capital was moved to Concord in 1808.

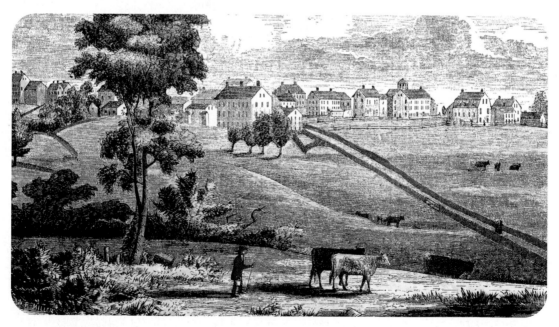

A New Hampshire village shown in the 1850s.

New Hampshire in the Civil War

Most people in New Hampshire were bitterly opposed to slavery. A New Hampshirite, "Honest John" Dickson of Keene, was the first person to speak out against slavery in the United States Congress, in 1835.

However, many people in New Hampshire were afraid the fight over slavery would cause the country to break up. One of them was Daniel Webster, a statesman and public speaker. He arranged the Compromise of 1850, between the "free" Northern states and the "slave" states of the South. This was an attempt to persuade the South to remain a part of the country. The compromise allowed slavery in some of the new states and territories in the West.

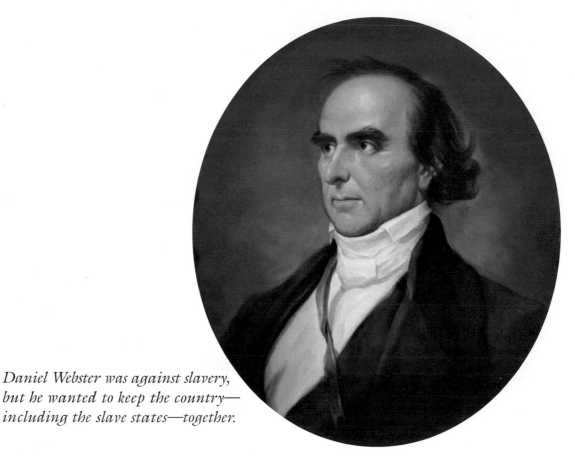

Daniel Webster was against slavery, but he wanted to keep the country—including the slave states—together.

Another politician who tried to find a peaceful solution was Franklin Pierce. He served as president of the United States from 1853 to 1857 and was the only New Hampshirite ever to become president. But all these efforts to maintain peace between the North and the South failed. Beginning in 1861, the United States was torn apart by the Civil War.

More than 39,000 soldiers from New Hampshire—almost half the men in the state—fought in the Civil War. At least 3,400 of them died, including a young man many people believed was the first Northern soldier to be killed in battle: Luther C. Ladd, from the little town of Alexandria.

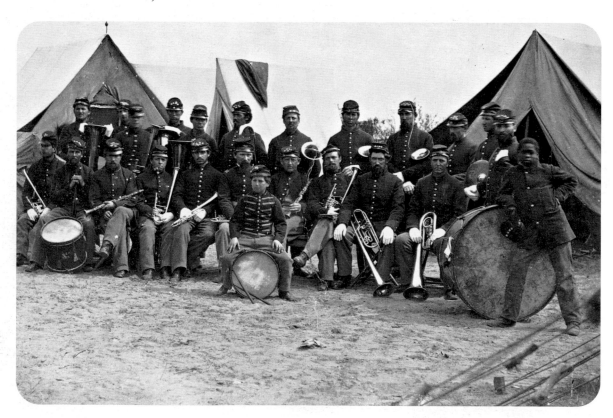

A New Hampshire Infantry Military Band at their camp in Hilton Head, South Carolina, during the Civil War.

When the Civil War ended, in 1865, New Hampshire's soldiers came home to a state that was changing fast. Factories and mills were replacing the family farms of New Hampshire. By the mid-1870s, more than half the workers in the state held manufacturing jobs, and the state was producing everything from shoes to window glass to pianos.

The 1860s were the only time when New Hampshire's population decreased. One reason was the number of people who died in the war. But people were also leaving to settle the new frontier territories. They were following the famous advice of Horace Greeley, a newspaper publisher from New Hampshire: "Go west, young man, and grow up with the country."

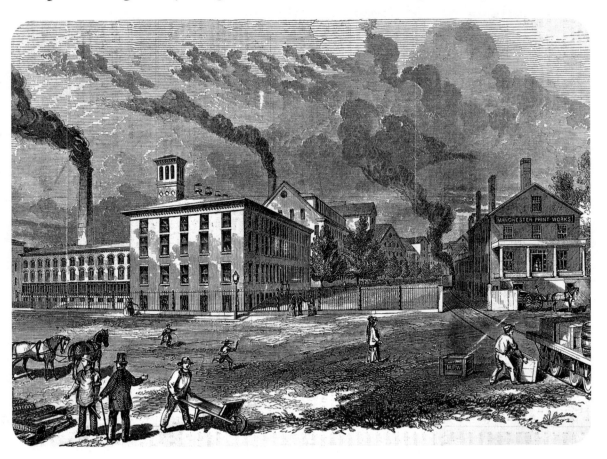

The Manchester Print Works in the mid 1800s.

One of New Hampshire's most important industries was textile (cloth) manufacturing. The largest textile mill in the world was the one built by the Amoskeag Manufacturing Company in Manchester. In the early 1900s, Amoskeag employed about 17,000 men, women, and children.

The mills and factories of New Hampshire needed more workers, and many immigrants began arriving, from as far away as Europe and as close by as Canada. So many immigrants came that by 1900, two out of every five New Hampshirites were immigrants or the children of immigrants.

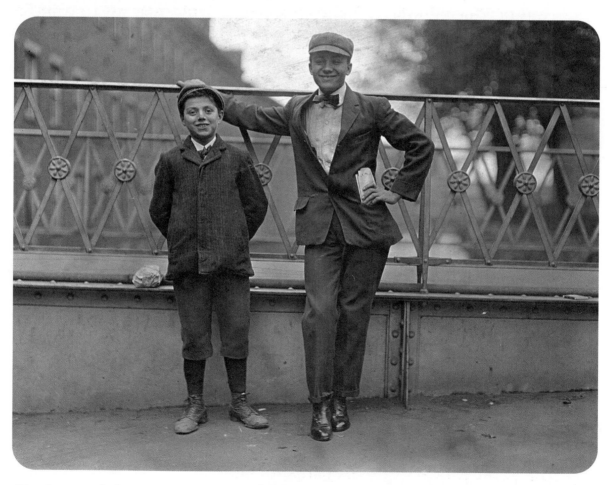

Two boys on their way to work the night shift at Amoskeag in 1909.

The White Mountains were beginning to open up, too. The railroad companies laid tracks into the mountains, to haul out lumber and paper from the saw mills and pulp mills of towns like Berlin. The same trains brought in a new resource: tourists. They came to visit the new resort hotels that were being built, and to try a winter sport Americans had just discovered: skiing.

Some of these visitors liked the state so much, they moved there. The state's population slowly increased.

In the early years of the twentieth century, New Hampshire hosted a peace conference that ended a war on the other side of the world. Signed on September 5, 1905, the Treaty of Portsmouth—which was actually signed at Wentworth by the Sea, an elegant hotel on nearby New Castle Island—ended a two-year conflict between Russia and Japan.

Modern Times

When the United States entered World War I, in 1917, New Hampshire's industry made an important contribution to the war effort. The state produced uniforms, shoes, weapons, and ships-especially submarines, which were then a new invention-for America's armed forces.

However, the time after World War I was difficult for New Hampshire. The textile industry was hit hard by competition from southern states. Then, in 1929, the Great Depression began. During the Depression, which lasted through the 1930s, New Hampshire-along with the rest of the country—suffered from poverty and unemployment. These problems were made even worse by natural disasters, including a terrible flood in 1936 and a hurricane in 1938. By the mid-1930s, even the great Amoskeag mills had shut down.

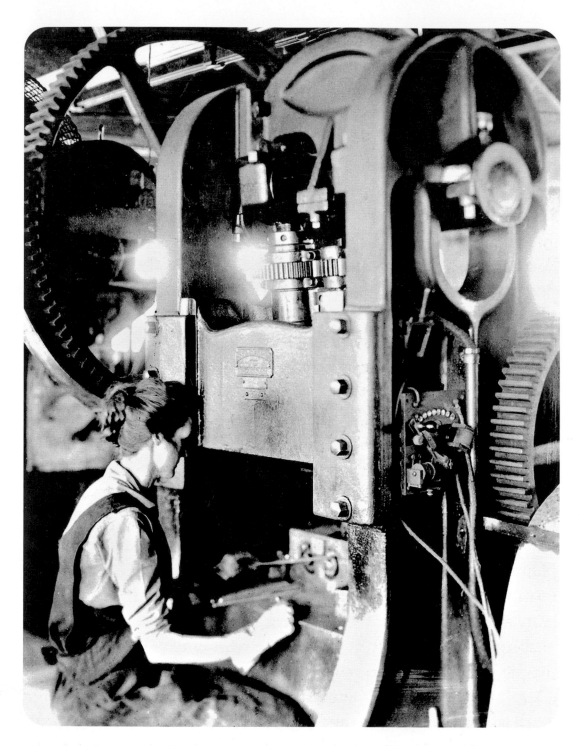

During the two World Wars, women worked in New Hampshire's factories and shipyards.

New Hampshire

World War II helped revive the state's industry. The shipyards of Portsmouth built submarines. Sometimes as many as two a week were built, and more than twenty thousand people found jobs at the shipyards. Many of the shipyard workers were women, because thousands of New Hampshire's men were serving in the armed forces.

Even during the war, New Hampshire was doing its part to create peace and prosperity. In 1944, government officials from all over the world gathered in the White Mountains, at the Bretton Woods resort, to create a new financial system for the postwar world. The result was the International Monetary Fund and the World Bank. These are still the foundations of the international economy.

The years after the war were also a time of change in New Hampshire. The state was growing as new types of industry arrived, drawn by skilled workers and low taxes. In the 1950s, small manufacturing companies—often making electronic equipment— began to take the place of textile mills and shoe factories. By the 1970s, "high-tech" companies, such as computer manufacturers, were becoming an important part of the state's economy.

These changes have not always been easy for the people of New Hampshire, who sometimes wonder whether their state is changing too fast. In the early 1970s, for example, a power company announced that it was planning to build a nuclear reactor at Seabrook, on the Atlantic Coast, to generate electricity. Some people in the state wanted the reactor built, to supply electrical energy for homes and businesses. But many others believed the reactor was dangerous and might damage the environment. Despite a political and legal battle that lasted seventeen years, the Seabrook nuclear reactor began producing electricity in 1990.

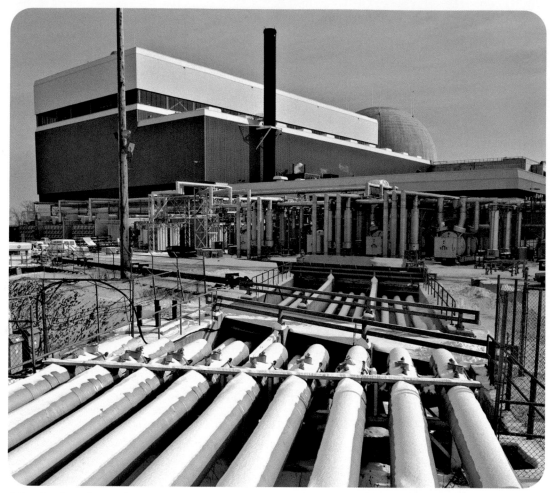

The Seabrook nuclear power plant produces more than half of the electricity generated in New Hampshire.

As New Hampshire enters the twenty-first century, the same concerns that made the struggle over Seabrook so bitter are still on New Hampshirites' minds. People want jobs and other economic benefits that come with progress, but they also want to preserve what they love best about their state. This problem—the need to balance old and new—has been the most important issue in New Hampshire for many years, and it will be for many years to come.

Important Dates

Around 8000 B.C.E. The area that will become New Hampshire is first occupied by Native Americans.

1614 John Smith explores the mouth of the Piscataqua River and the Isles of Shoals.

1622 Captain George Mason and Sir Ferdinando Gorges are given a huge tract of land in New England.

1623 English colonists establish a settlement called Pannaway Plantation, near the present-day town of Rye.

1629 Mason and Gorges divide their land, and Mason names his section New Hampshire.

John Smith

1689–1763 The French and Indian Wars begin with a Native American attack on Dover, New Hampshire.

1774 A raid on the British fort on New Castle Island marks the first armed conflict of the Revolutionary War.

1784 New Hampshire becomes the first colony to create its own independent government.

1788 New Hampshire becomes the ninth state.

1808 The state capital is moved from Portsmouth to Concord.

1853 Franklin Pierce, a native of Exeter, is sworn in as the fourteenth president of the United States.

1864 Salmon P. Chase of Cornish becomes chief justice of the United States Supreme Court.

1905 The Treaty of Portsmouth ends the Russo-Japanese War.

1936 The Amoskeag mills in Manchester end most production.

1944 The Bretton Woods Conference creates the world's new financial system.

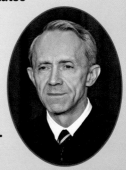

1961 Alan B. Shephard of East Derry becomes the first American in space.

1990 David Souter of New Hampshire is appointed to the United States Supreme Court.

David Souter

2001 The United States Supreme Court settles a longstanding "border" dispute by granting the Portsmouth Naval Shipyard—long claimed by New Hampshire—to the state of Maine.

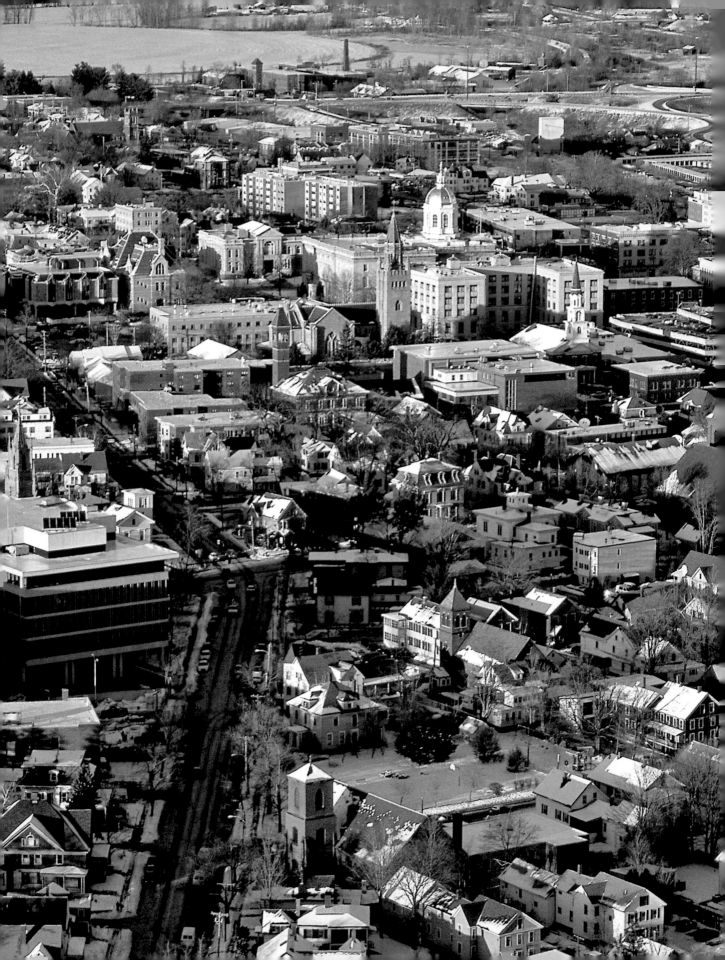

3 The People

Until the Europeans began exploring the region in the 1600s, Native Americans were the only people to live on the land now known as New Hampshire. For more than two hundred years after the start of exploration, most New Hampshirites were typical New England "Yankees"—people of English or Scottish ancestry. But in the mid-1800s, the makeup of the state and its people began to change a great deal.

Immigrants were flooding into New Hampshire, to work in the state's fast-growing factories and mills. They came from Ireland, Germany, Scandinavia, Poland, Greece, and other parts of Europe. But the new arrivals who had the greatest impact on New Hampshire came from right next door: the Canadian province of Quebec.

These immigrants spoke French, and were mostly Roman Catholic. Although they were drawn to the economic opportunity New Hampshire offered, they were determined to preserve their language, their religion, and their culture. They succeeded. Today, almost one-quarter of the people of New Hampshire

Concord, the capital of the state, seen from the air.

are of French-Canadian ancestry, and the French Canadians have left their mark everywhere in the state. Paul Tardiff, a schoolteacher in Berlin, remembers that when he was a child, in the 1940s, "just about the only language you'd hear on the street was French." The French language had declined somewhat by the 1970s, but Tardiff says that it has made a comeback since then. "The kids here are studying the language in school, and they're keeping their culture and traditions alive."

The first French-Canadians who came to New Hampshire often chose to live in separate areas, called *petits Canadas* (little Canadas), with their own French-language schools, churches, and businesses. Today, people of French-Canadian ancestry are much more a part of the daily life of the state. But as many as 60,000 New Hampshirites still say that French is their native language.

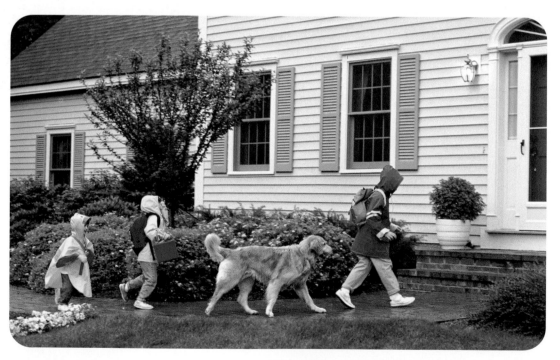

Many people move to—and stay in—New Hampshire because of the excellent neighborhoods and schools.

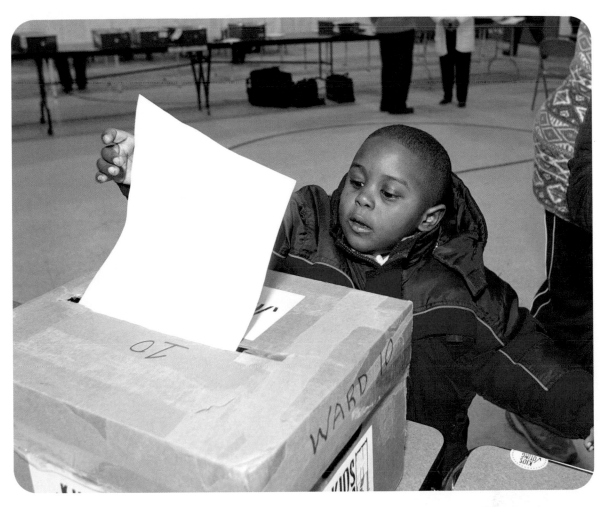

A young New Hampshirite takes part in elections at a school in his neighborhood.

New Hampshire is still less diverse, ethnically and culturally, than most states. About 98 percent of New Hampshirites are Caucasian, or white, and only about 8 percent speak a language other than English at home. But the state continues to grow and change.

People from other states—and from other countries—are bringing their influences to New Hampshire. Some new residents are people from other states who had visited or attended school in New Hampshire, and later decided to move there.

The People

Others move to the state to enjoy its peaceful surroundings. Claudio Marcus, who moved to the United States from the South American nation of Chile when he was twelve, is one of those people. In 2000, he and his wife left the big city of Baltimore, Maryland, to settle in the small New Hampshire village of Andover. "We came here looking for the things everybody wants," he says. "Good schools, safe neighborhoods, a great place for our kids to grow up. And we definitely found those things here." If he had any doubts about being welcomed in a state with few Spanish-speaking residents, they went away quickly. "We'd only been here a few weeks when one of our new neighbors invited us to our first town meeting."

Cities and Towns

One reason that New Hampshire is able to keep its traditional neighborly spirit is that most people live in small, close-knit population centers. The three largest cities in New Hampshire—

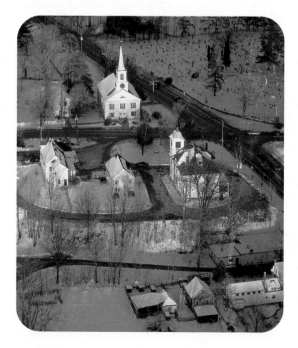

Manchester, Nashua, and Concord—have a combined population of only a little more than 200,000. And most New Hampshirites live in even smaller towns, in tiny villages, and in the countryside. Many residents make their homes in communities where their families have lived for generations.

Some believe that this neighborly spirit might soon disappear. Many

A small village near Manchester.

people now commute from Portsmouth and the other towns of the Seacoast to jobs in the Boston area, which is an hour's drive to the south. Others now "telecommute"—using technologies such as e-mail and the Internet to work from their homes. The result, some longtime New Hampshirites complain, is that the Seacoast is becoming just another suburb of Boston.

But the Seacoast—and the rest of New Hampshire—are very much as they have always been. Even though many of the state's cities and towns now have the same shopping malls and fast-food restaurants as the rest of America, they remain, for the most part, quiet and peaceful. There is a good reason: That is the way almost everyone—longtime residents and visitors alike—wants New Hampshire to stay.

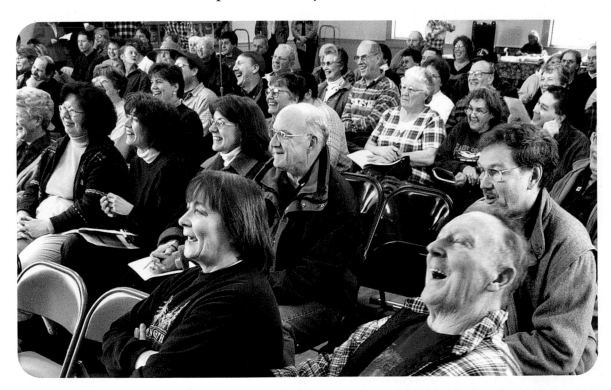

New Hampshirites meet at community meetings to discuss issues that are important to them.

Famous New Hampshirites

Jeanne Shaheen: Politician

Jeanne Shaheen was the first woman to serve as governor of New Hampshire. She was born in St. Charles, Missouri, but moved to New Hampshire and became a high school teacher and then a businesswoman. She was elected to the governor's office three times—in 1996, 1998, and 2000. As a former teacher, she gave her greatest attention to issues that affect children, such as school standards and health care.

Passaconnaway: Native American Leader

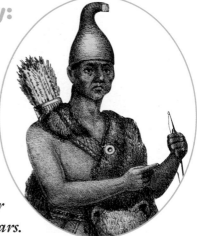

Passaconnaway, a great chief of the Pennacook group, believed his people should not fight with the European settlers. In a famous speech, he said the Great Spirit of the Pennacook had told him, "Tell your people. Peace, Peace, is the only hope of your race." The treaty he arranged in 1644—known as "the Peace of Passaconnaway"—kept New Hampshire's Native Americans from going to war for almost fifty years.

Alan Shepard: Astronaut

Alan Shepard, born in East Derry, New Hampshire, was the first American in space. He served as a naval officer in World War II, then became a test pilot and later an astronaut. On May 5, 1961, his space capsule, Freedom 7, was launched from Cape Canaveral in Florida, for a fifteen-minute flight that reached a height of 115 miles. Ten years later, on the Apollo 14 expedition, Shepard walked on the surface of the moon.

Robert Frost: Poet

Robert Frost was born in San Francisco, but lived most of his working life in New Hampshire, and wrote more than half of his poems there. "It has been New Hampshire with me all the way," he once said. "You will find my poems show it, I think." The Robert Frost Farm near Derry, where he lived until his death in 1963, is now a popular destination for visitors.

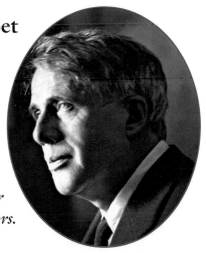

Franklin Pierce: President of the United States

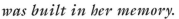

Franklin Pierce, born in Hillsboro, was the fourteenth president of the United States. He served as president from 1853 to 1857. Though he had been a respected congressman and senator, as president he became very unpopular in many parts of the country—partly because he tried to reach a compromise over the issue of slavery.

Christa McAuliffe: Teacher and Astronaut

Christa McAuliffe, who taught social studies at Concord High School, was chosen from among 11,500 applicants to be the first civilian (a person who is not in the military) in space. On January 28, 1986, she took off on the space shuttle Challenger *from the Kennedy Space Center in Florida. Just seventy-three seconds later, the shuttle exploded, killing everyone on board. The Christa McAuliffe Planetarium in Concord was built in her memory.*

Fun in New Hampshire

The people of New Hampshire are very interested in preserving the state's special traditions. You can see that at the many summer festivals and fall fairs that celebrate New Hampshire's old small-town ways, and in the historic monuments, museums, and Revolutionary War celebrations that attract visitors to the state. And you can see it, too, in New Hampshire's centuries-old love of the arts.

Since 1907, the MacDowell Colony, an artists' retreat near Peterborough founded by the composer Edward MacDowell, has offered writers, painters, and composers from all over the country a quiet place to create art. While staying at the MacDowell Colony, Thornton Wilder wrote his famous play *Our Town*, which depicts New Hampshire life in the early 1900s.

New Hampshire has welcomed writers, painters, and other artists for many years. Among the creative people who have lived in the Granite State are Robert Frost, the novelists J. D. Salinger, and John Irving, and the sculptors Daniel Chester French and Augustus Saint-Gaudens.

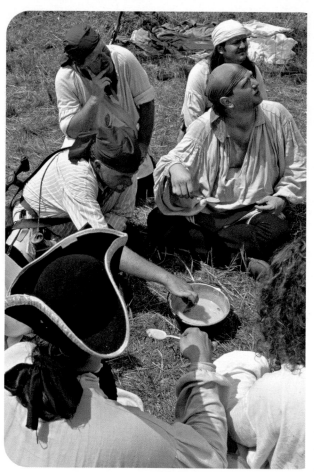

A historical reenactment honors New Hampshire's past.

What do most New Hampshirites have in common? More than anything, it is a deep love of New Hampshire and its history, traditions, and customs. The people of New Hampshire—both longtime residents and newcomers—know they live in a very special place. And they will always work to celebrate the things that make it so special. After all, that is why most of them came to the New Hampshire in the first place.

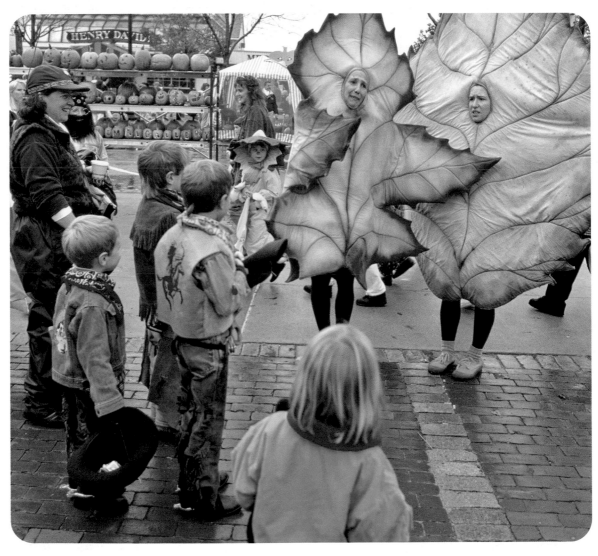

Residents take part in a harvest festival in Keene.

The People

Calendar of Events

Frostbite Follies Winter Carnival

Every February, Bethlehem and many of the neighboring towns in the White Mountains celebrate the joys of a New Hampshire winter. Activities include cross-country skiing, snowshoeing, and sleigh rides.

Annual Wildquack River Festival

This one-day event, held in May on the Wildcat River, in the White Mountain town of Jackson, may be the biggest annual rubber-duck race in the world. (Of course, it may also be the *only* annual rubber-duck race in the world.) Thousands of rubber ducks float down the river and over Jackson Falls, competing for the title of fastest, noisiest, or most unique duck in the race.

Somersworth International Children's Festival

This big festival, held in June every year, attracts kids of all ages with music and crafts, animals and games.

Festival du Bois

In July, the north-country town of Berlin celebrates its past with French-Canadian crafts and a re-creation of a nineteenth-century logging camp. One of the highlights every year is a traditional "bean hole supper," where the beans are cooked in a big hole in the ground.

Hillsborough Balloon Festival

Every July, the skies above the little town of Hillsborough are filled with brightly colored hot-air balloons. New Hampshirites and people from neighboring states go up in the air to enjoy the amazing view.

The Coleville Annual North Country Moose Festival

Exeter Revolutionary War Festival

The seacoast town of Exeter celebrates the American Revolution in July, with eighteenth-century costumes and music, and a reenactment of an actual Revolutionary War battle.

League of New Hampshire Craftsmen's Fair

For more than seventy years, the craftspeople of New Hampshire have been showing their best work—jewelry, pottery, woodworking, and much more—at this annual fair, now held in Newbury in August.

New Hampshire Highland Games

Every September, this colorful event, now held at the Hopkinton State Fairgrounds, celebrates all things Scottish—from kilts and tartans to bagpipes and fiddles.

White Mountain Central Railroad Days

If you love steam engines, Lincoln is the place to be in September. You can see and ride some of the historic trains that have traveled all over the state since the 1800s.

Deerfield Fair

The oldest event of its kind in New England, this agricultural fair, held in late September, has been featuring livestock shows, sheepdog trials, and many other traditional rural events since 1876.

Apple Harvest Day

This delicious festival, held in Dover in early October, celebrates one of New Hampshire's best-known agricultural products with apples, apples, and more apples.

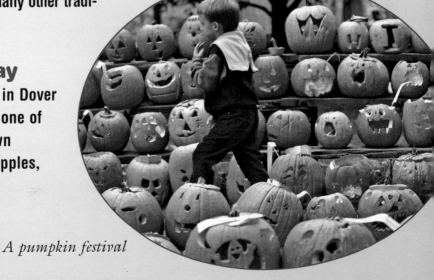

A pumpkin festival

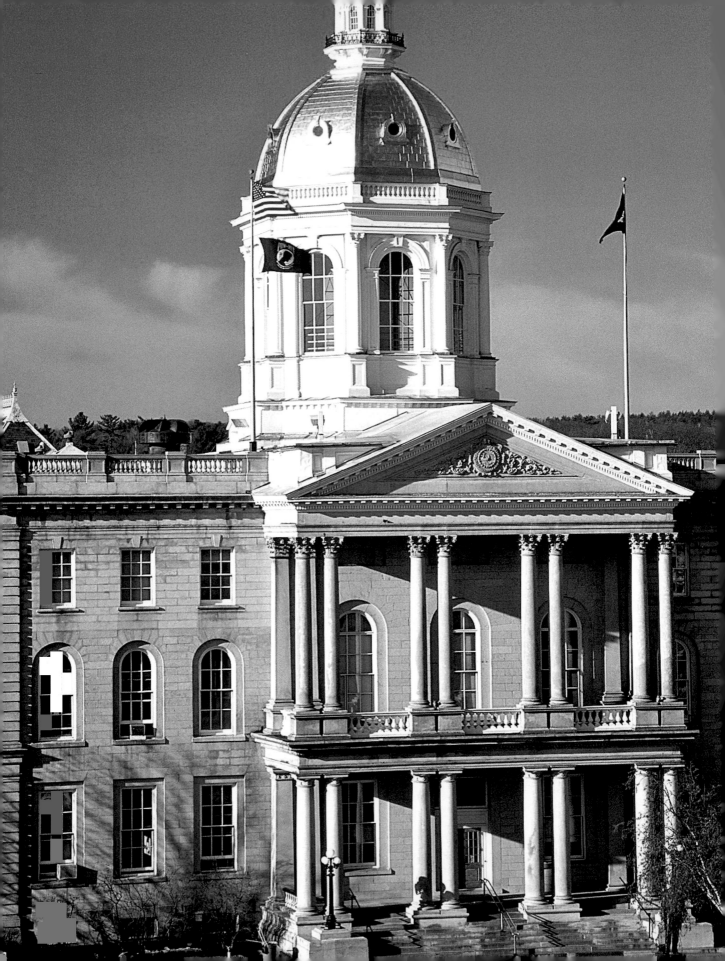

4 How It Works

Every four years, in the middle of the bitterly cold New Hampshire winter, the entire nation's attention is focused on this small state. Politicians walk the snowy streets of New Hampshire's cities and towns—often followed by newspaper reporters and television crews. They shake hands with every voter they can find. Why? The politicians are running for president, and the New Hampshire primary, as this voting event is called, is the starting point of every presidential election.

The two main political parties—Democratic and Republican—use the state primaries to choose the candidates who will run in the presidential election the following November. Many states have primaries, but New Hampshire's is always the first, and many people believe it is the most important.

The New Hampshire primary was originally scheduled for May. Many farmers found it hard to come in to town to vote at that time of year, because they were busy plowing their fields and planting crops. So in 1915, the primary was moved to its now-traditional date: the second Tuesday in March. The first New Hampshire primary took place on March 9, 1920.

The New Hampshire state capitol in Concord.

New Hampshire has representatives at the federal, or national, level. Two senators are elected, by all the voters of the state, to serve six-year terms in Washington, D.C. Two members of the United States House of Representatives are elected—one from each of the state's two congressional districts—to serve two-year terms.

Branches of Government

The state government is divided into three branches

Executive The governor is the head of the executive branch. This branch carries out the laws passed by the legislative branch, but he or she shares power with a five-member executive council. The governor and the executive council are elected to two-year terms in statewide elections.

Legislative New Hampshire's legislature is called the General Court. It has two parts: the senate, with twenty-four members; and the house of representatives, with four hundred members. (The New Hampshire house of representatives is the largest state legislature in the country, and one of the largest in the world.) The members of the General Court, who are elected for two-year terms, pass the laws and regulations that govern New Hampshire.

Judicial New Hampshire's judges are appointed by the governor, and serve until they reach the retirement age of seventy. The state supreme court—the highest court in New Hampshire—has one chief justice and four associate justices. Presently, the New Hampshire superior court has twenty-seven justices.

The people of New Hampshire take national politics very seriously, but it is at the state and local levels that they really get involved. This means that most of them also have to have regular jobs. By doing so, they are able to keep in close touch with the concerns of "regular folks."

New Hampshire politics gets really interesting at the local level. The heart and soul of local politics in the state is the centuries-old tradition of the town meeting. This is one of the purest forms of "direct democracy" in the world. Direct democracy means that the people themselves—not just their elected representatives—vote on important issues.

The state has 221 communities, called "towns," and most of the towns hold an annual town meeting. Every single one of the town's voters can come to the meeting, speak his or her mind, and then vote on the issue. "This is everyone's chance to be heard," says Linda Hall, deputy town clerk of Merrimack. "I don't think there's anyone here who would ever be willing to give up the town meeting."

The rest of the year, the town is run by a group of three to five elected representatives called selectmen (even though they can be either men or women), who are elected to three-year terms. But all the big decisions about how the town will be run—from who gets the

The first New Hampshire legislature met at this meeting house in Concord.

snowplowing contract to how the schools will be paid for—are made at the town meeting.

One of the most important political issues in New Hampshire, year after year, is taxation. Most states have a state income tax, a state sales tax or both. The money collected from these taxes pays for the state's expenses. But New Hampshire has neither a sales tax nor an income tax. That leaves the state with a big problem that never seems to go away: how to pay for the services that governments, both state and local, provide for their citizens.

Education for the state's children is one of the most important of those services. The schools in the state are under the control of the towns, and their quality varies widely from one town to the next. The schools in the wealthier towns have many extras such as computers and after-school athletic programs. But towns with less money cannot afford such extras. In 1997, the New Hampshire Supreme Court ruled that this situation was unfair, and said the state government had to give an equally good education to all students, no matter where they lived. Unfortunately, the court did not say where the money to pay for it was going to come from. In the years since the court's ruling, the state government has struggled to find ways to come up with the money. Many ideas have been suggested—including a statewide income tax and property tax—but nobody has yet found a solution that all the people of New Hampshire can agree on.

How You Can Make a Difference

New Hampshire's tradition of direct participation in politics makes it easy to get involved. Even if you are not old enough to officially vote, you can attend your town meeting and watch your fellow citizens make decisions. Another way to learn about

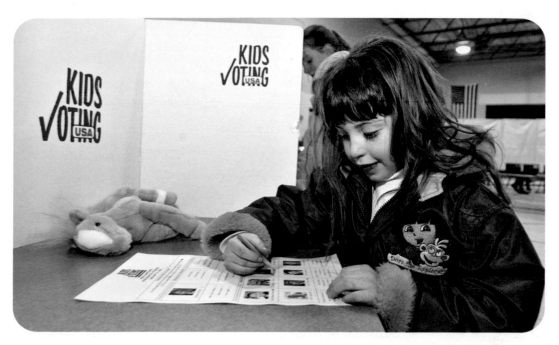

This Manchester student is choosing a presidential candidate in the New Hampshire primary.

the democratic process is to participate in Kids Voting USA. This unique program gives children a chance to learn about their political system and "vote" for the candidates they think will do the best job. To learn more, visit http://www.kidsvotingusa.org/intro/overview.asp. You can also attend sessions of both houses of the state legislature, and even watch your senators and your representative at work in Washington, D.C.

If there is an issue you care about, you should definitely get involved. Figure out who you need to talk to, then write a letter, make a telephone call, or send an e-mail message. You can make a difference.

To find your state legislators, visit this Web site:
http://www.gencourt.state.nh.us/ie/whosmyleg
You will need to know the county and town you live in. If you are not sure, ask a parent, teacher, or librarian to help you.

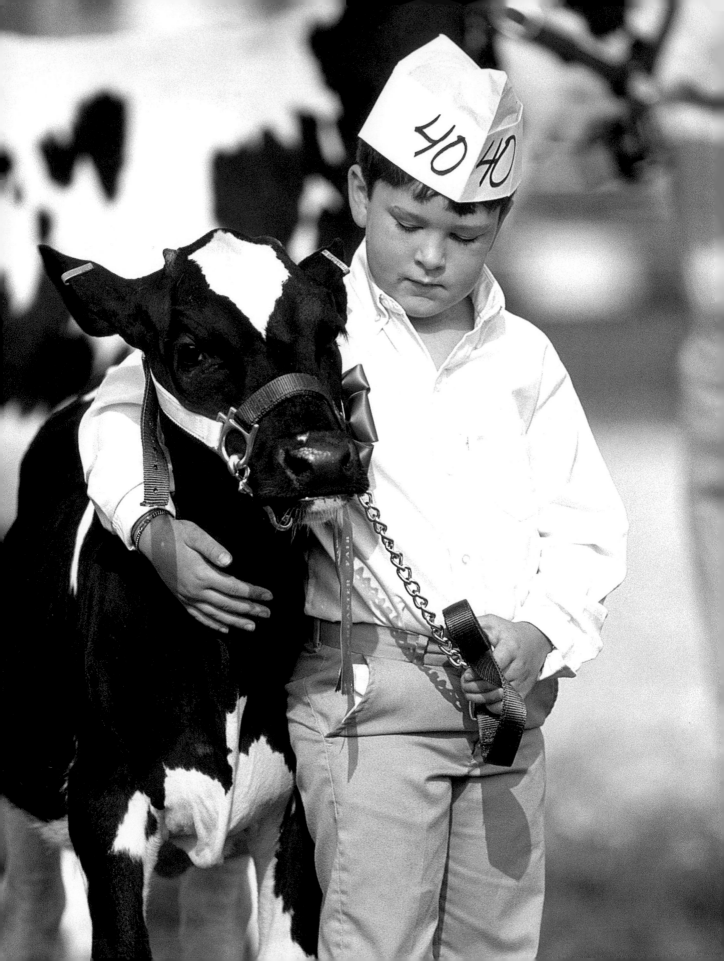

5 Making a Living

The people of New Hampshire have always worked hard. But the ways they make their living have changed a lot in recent years. Many of the traditional New Hampshire industries are now far less important to the state's economy than they once were.

New Hampshire is still known as the Granite state, but granite quarrying no longer employs very many people. The main reason is that concrete, steel, and other modern building materials have replaced granite in most construction products.

Farming—the backbone of the New Hampshire economy until the mid-1800s—has also declined in importance. The state still has more than three thousand farms, but they account for only about 1 percent of its economic activity. New Hampshire farms produce dairy products and grow crops such as hay and potatoes. Farmers across the state also grow fruits such as apples, blueberries, and strawberries. There are also dozens of farms raising livestock, including cows, sheep, and horses.

A young New Hampshirite shows his cow at a country fair in Lancaster.

Recipe for Apple Turnovers

Here is a delicious variation on a traditional recipe from the Granite State. Cortland and Northern Spy apples—two types of apple that grow in New Hampshire—will work especially well.

Ingredients:

8-ounce package of frozen puff pastry (thawed according to package directions)

2 large apples, peeled, cored, and cut into pieces

1/4 cup sugar

1/4 teaspoon apple pie spice (or allspice, or a combination of cinnamon and nutmeg)

3 tablespoons butter

1 egg (beaten) for glazing

1 tablespoon sugar

Have an adult help you with the oven and preheat it to 400 degrees. Using a rolling pin, roll the pastry into a 12" x 18" rectangle, then cut it into 6 squares and place it on a baking sheet.

In a bowl, combine the apples, the 1/4 cup of sugar, and the spices. Divide the mixture evenly among the pastry squares and dot with butter. Moisten the edges of the pastry squares with water, then fold each one over diagonally to form a triangle. Press down on the edges with your fingers, and then seal them with a fork. Using the fork, make a few holes in each triangle.

Brush the triangles with the beaten-egg glaze, and sprinkle them with the remaining sugar. Bake in the oven for 20 minutes or until the pasty turns golden.

Remove the turnovers from the oven and place them on a rack to cool. Watch your fingers when the turnovers come out of the oven because they will be very hot. When the turnovers have cooled, you can eat them plain or with a scoop of ice cream.

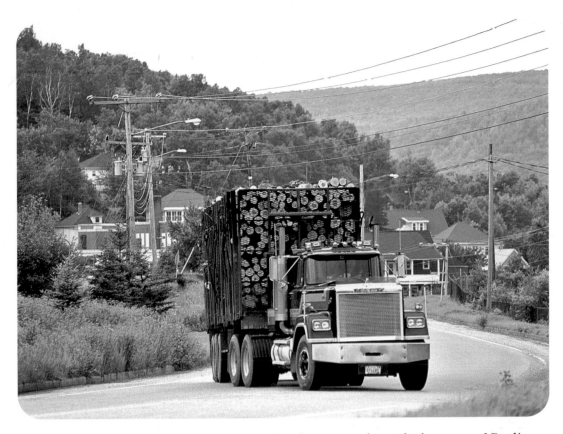

A truck loaded with New Hampshire lumber passes through the town of Berlin.

Some of the old ways of making a living remain, however. The timber industry is heavily concentrated in the northern part of the state. Thousands of New Hampshirites work for lumber companies. They cut down trees, haul them to mills, and turn them into everything from plywood to paper.

The Portsmouth Naval Shipyard has been building and repairing warships—from clipper ships to nuclear submarines—for more than two centuries. The shipyard is still in business, but it is not in New Hampshire anymore. On May 29, 2001, the United States Supreme Court settled a centuries-old boundary dispute by moving the state line—and placing the historic shipyard in Maine.

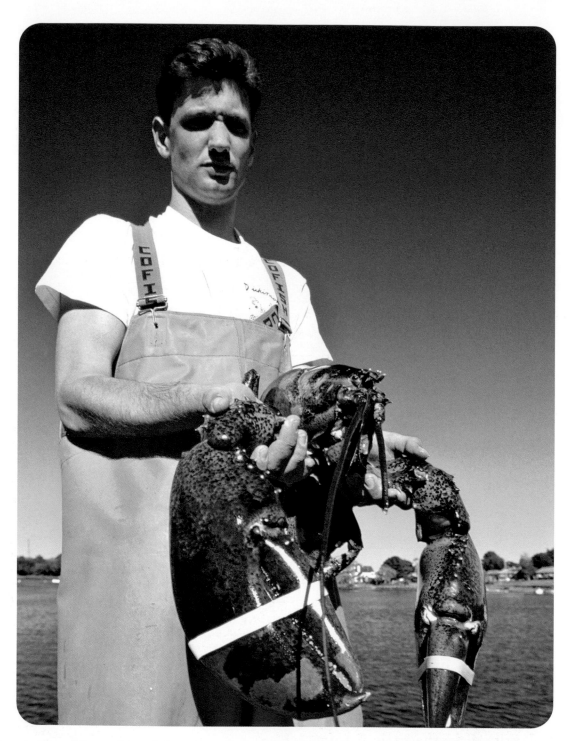

A New Hampshire fisherman shows off a live lobster he has just caught. If the lobster's claws were not banded, the fisherman could lose his fingers.

New Hampshire

New Hampshire still makes the most of its short coastline, too, just as it has since the days of Pannaway Plantation. The state's small but valuable fishing industry hauls in cod, flounder, haddock, lobster, and shrimp. The seacoast town of Portsmouth is still an important international seaport, handling hundreds of thousands of tons of shipping every year.

Manufacturing

The New Hampshire economy depends very heavily on manufacturing, just as it has for more than a century. The manufacturing industry is the second-largest segment of the state's economy, employing more than 80,000 people. Many of the products these workers make are traditional New Hampshire specialties, such as clothing and leather goods. The state also produces everything from machine tools to plastics and chemicals.

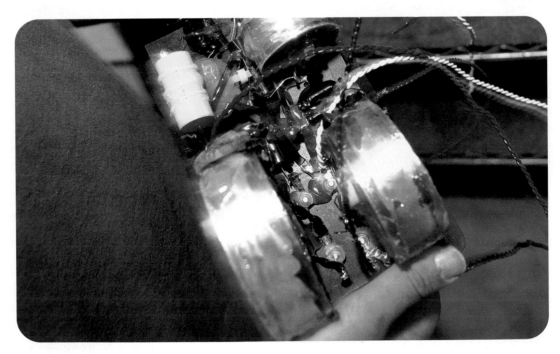

A designer works on a loudspeaker at a factory in New Hampshire.

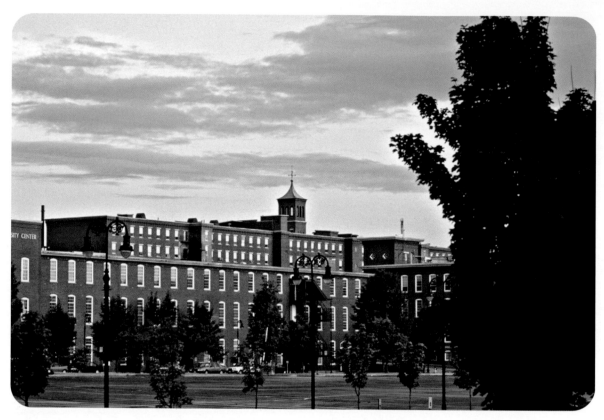

The buildings that once housed the Amoskeag mills in Manchester.

The huge Amoskeag mill buildings in Manchester were abandoned for years, but now they are home to manufacturing plants, software companies, museums, art galleries, and restaurants. Dennis Delay, an economist in Manchester, says, "The revival of Amoskeag shows just what the people of New Hampshire can achieve when they put their minds to it."

More and more, however, New Hampshire's manufacturing industry is built on technology. The high-tech trend began in the 1970s, when computer manufacturers started moving into the state, attracted by skilled workers, good working and living conditions, and low taxes. By 2000, New Hampshire was truly a high-tech state, with more than 8 percent of its workers in

New Hampshire

technology-related jobs. That is even more than in California, the center of the world's computer industry. Today, New Hampshire companies make computer components, telecommunications equipment, software, scientific instruments, medical devices, and many other highly advanced products.

One of the most interesting of the state's high-tech products is the Segway Human Transporter, a two-wheeled, self-balancing, electric-powered "people mover." It has already conquered New Hampshire's highest peak. On August 28, 2003, a Segway climbed Mount Washington. It took two and a half hours, three riders, and six sets of batteries, but the Segway finally made it up all 7.6 miles of very steep, not-always-paved roads

The state also encourages its young residents to become interested in technology. In 1992, Dean Kamen of Manchester created the FIRST Robotics Competition, which is designed to create awareness of science and technology among young people. FIRST teams—which include high school and college students and industry experts—design and build advanced robots. From its beginning in a Manchester school gym, the competition has grown to include hundreds of teams from all over the world.

New Hampshire's "tech-friendly" environment is also drawing some of the best scientific minds in the country. Dr. Charles Brenner, a leading cancer researcher, moved his entire genetics laboratory from Philadelphia to the little town of Lebanon in 2003. "New Hampshire offers me all the facilities I need for my work," he says, "and the quality of life here makes it possible to attract first-class research staff."

Products & Resources

Trees

About 4.8 million acres—84 percent of New Hampshire's land area—is covered by trees. The state's hardwood trees, such as ash, birch, and oak, are used for lumber for construction. Softwoods, like pine and spruce, are sent to paper mills. New Hampshire even produces many of the nation's Christmas trees.

Biotechnology

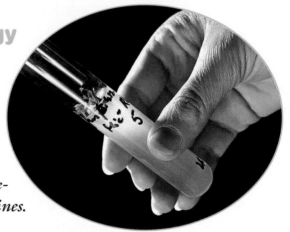

One of New Hampshire's fastest-growing industries is biotechnology, which involves finding new uses for living organisms. Many New Hampshire companies, most of them located along the seacoast, are doing advanced biotechnology research, which is especially important in developing new medicines.

Computer Software

So many software companies are located in the state that New Hampshire has been called "the silicon state." (Silicon is an element used in computer parts.) Computer-aided design, Internet security, and desktop publishing are just a few of the Granite State's software specialties.

Leather Products

New Hampshirites have been skilled at making animal hides into fine leather goods since colonial times. The state's first shoe factory opened in Weare in 1823, and leather manufacturing is still a very important industry there. New Hampshire's leather manufacturers exported $185 million worth of leather goods in 2000.

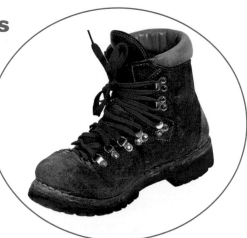

Potatoes

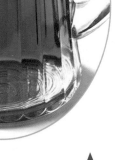

New Hampshire is not as well known for growing potatoes as neighboring Maine. But the first potato in the United States was planted in Londonderry, New Hampshire, in 1719. There are still many potato farms in the state, especially in the western part of the White Mountains region.

Maple Syrup

New Hampshire's maple syrup season is short—just a few weeks in March and April—but very sweet. Every year, the state's maple trees produce about 90,000 gallons of syrup. That is pretty amazing, when you consider that it takes about forty gallons of tree sap to make just one gallon of syrup.

Service Industries

Despite the importance of industry—both high-tech and the more traditional kinds—most New Hampshirites actually make their living in service jobs. Doctors, lawyers, salesclerks, and real estate agents perform services for other people. The most important service industry in New Hampshire, and the second-largest part of the state's economy, is travel and tourism.

Each year, visitors bring billions of dollars into the state. Tourism employs more than 65,000 people. One of New Hampshire's most famous tourist attractions is its beautiful old covered bridges. More than fifty covered bridges can be found in the state. This includes the longest one in the country, the 460-foot Cornish-Windsor Bridge, built in 1866.

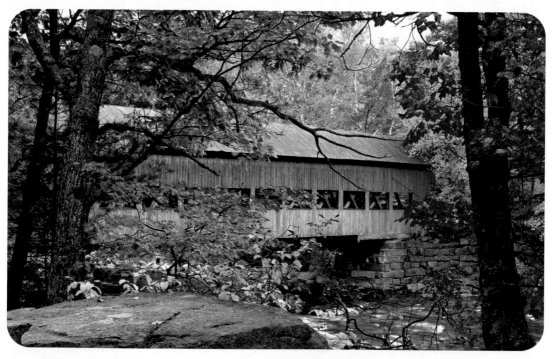

The Albany Bridge was first built over the Swift River in 1857, but was destroyed by a windstorm in 1858. The bridge was rebuilt, and through the years, parts of the bridge have been changed to keep it safe.

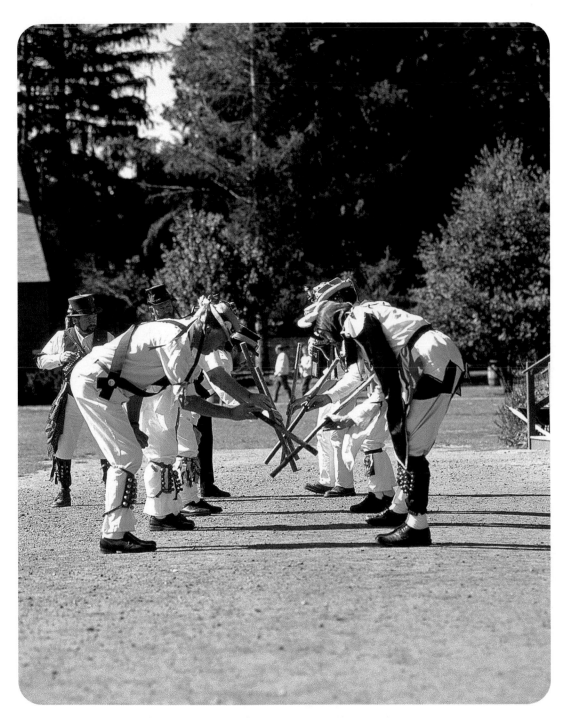

Throughout the year, visitors can watch reenactments and other presentations at the state's history museums. Museums and other tourist attractions provide jobs for many New Hampshirites.

Making a Living

It is easy to understand why so many people come to New Hampshire for their vacations. The state offers so many pleasures, from the beaches of the seacoast in the summertime to the ski slopes of the White Mountains in the winter. In fact, New Hampshire was the home of the first summer resort in America, in Wolfeboro. In 1767, John Wentworth, the colonial governor, built a summer home on the shores of the lake that now bears his name. Many other wealthy people did the same, and the first summer resort in America was born.

In the years since then, many people have followed in Governor Wentworth's footsteps, and have made New Hampshire one of the most popular tourist destinations in the United States. Every year, hundreds of thousands of people visit the beaches of the seacoast, the lakes and rivers of the Uplands, and the mountains and notches of the White Mountains. They come to visit the state's many summer festivals, admire the glorious autumn leaves, and enjoy the winter skiing in the White Mountains.

Most of all, they come because New Hampshirites offer them a warm welcome. In fact, you could say that the people of New Hampshire are the state's most valuable resource. With their love of tradition, their Yankee ingenuity, their passion for democracy, and their friendly ways, they make sure that New Hampshire remains one of the best places in the country to visit—and to live in.

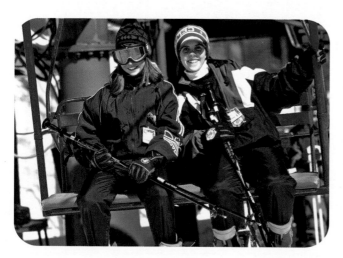

Two young skiers catch a lift up Wildcat Mountain.

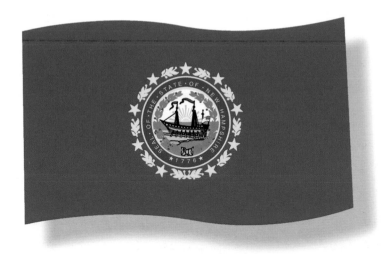

New Hampshire's state flag shows the state seal on a blue background. The seal is surrounded by laurel leaves—a traditional symbol of victory—and nine stars that show that New Hampshire is the ninth state.

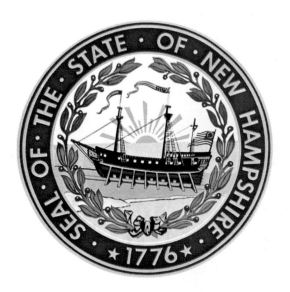

The state seal shows the frigate Raleigh—built in Portsmouth in 1776 for the new American navy—with a granite boulder in front and the rising sun behind. This scene is circled by laurel wreaths, the words Seal of the State of New Hampshire, and the date 1776.

NEW HAMPSHIRE

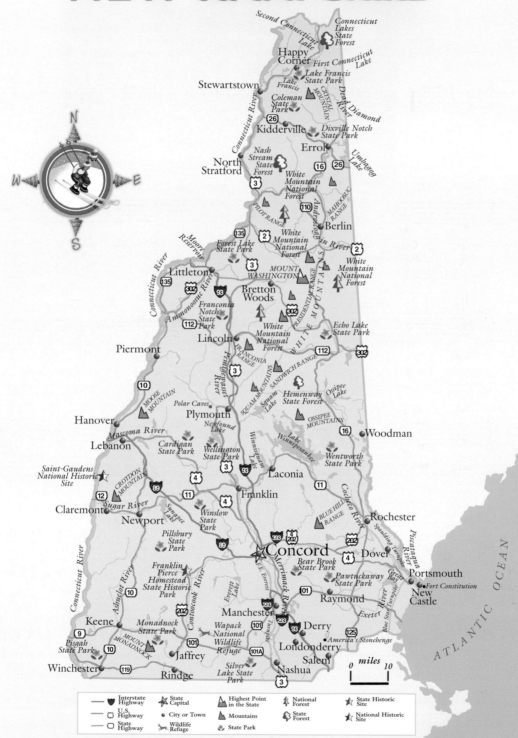

Second Connecticut Lake
Connecticut Lakes State Forest
Happy Corner
First Connecticut Lake
Stewartstown
Lake Francis State Park
Lake Francis
CRYSTAL MOUNTAIN
Dead Diamond River
Coleman State Park
26
Kidderville
Dixville Notch State Park
North Stratford
Errol
Umbagog Lake
Nash Stream State Forest
16
26
White Mountain National Forest
Connecticut River
3
PILOT RANGE
110
MAHOOSUC RANGE
Berlin
135
2
White Mountain National Forest
2
Forest Lake State Park
White Mountain National Forest
Moore Reservoir
3
MOUNT WASHINGTON
Littleton
135
Bretton Woods
93
302
PRESIDENTIAL RANGE
White Mountain National Forest
Ammonoosuc River
Franconia Notch State Park
302
Echo Lake State Park
112
Lincoln
White Mountain National Forest
302
WHITE MOUNTAINS
Piermont
FRANCONIA RANGE
112
SANDWICH RANGE
Pemigewasset River
SQUAM MOUNTAINS
Hemenway State Forest
Ossipee Lake
10
Squam Lake
MOOSE MOUNTAIN
Polar Caves
Plymouth
Newfound Lake
OSSIPEE MOUNTAINS
Hanover
Mascoma River
Lake Winnipesaukee
16
Woodman
Lebanon
Cardigan State Park
Wellington State Park
Wentworth State Park
Winnisquam Lake
3
93
Saint-Gaudens National Historic Site
CROYDON MOUNTAIN
4
Laconia
11
Cochero River
Rochester
12
89
11
Sugar River
4
Franklin
Claremont
Newport
Winslow State Park
BLUE HILLS RANGE
Spofford Lake
89
Dover
Pillsbury State Park
393
202
202
Concord
4
Ashuelot River
Bear Brook State Park
Portsmouth
Franklin Pierce Homestead State Historic Park
F.E. Everett Turnpike
Merrimack River
Pawtuckaway State Park
Great Bay
Fort Constitution
New Castle
202
Raymond
Exeter
01
Keene
Monadnock State Park
Contoocook River
Everett Lake
293
Manchester
255
Derry
America's Stonehenge
125
9
MOUNT MONADNOCK
101
Wapack National Wildlife Refuge
101
93
Londonderry
Pisgah State Park
10
Jaffrey
101A
Salem
Winchester
119
Rindge
Silver Lake State Park
Nashua
3

ATLANTIC OCEAN

miles
0   10

Legend

- Interstate Highway
- U.S. Highway
- State Highway
- State Capital
- City or Town
- Wildlife Refuge
- Highest Point in the State
- Mountains
- State Park
- National Forest
- State Forest
- State Historic Site
- National Historic Site

74

Old New Hampshire

Words by John Franklin Holmes
Music by Maurice Hoffmann

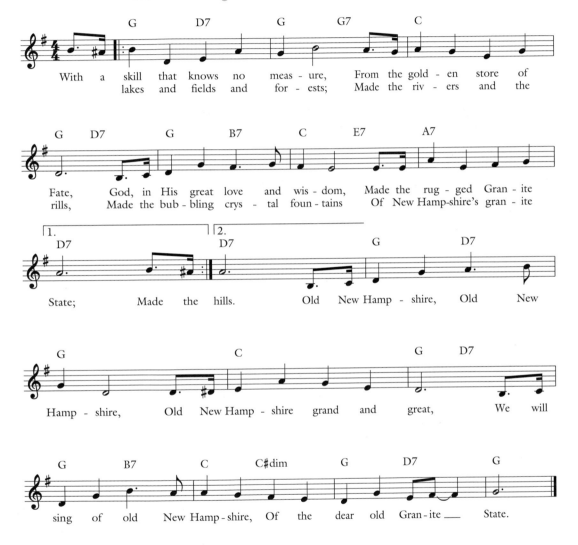

With a skill that knows no meas - ure, From the gold - en store of
lakes and fields and for - ests; Made the riv - ers and the

Fate, God, in His great love and wis - dom, Made the rug - ged Gran - ite
rills, Made the bub - bling crys - tal foun - tains Of New Hamp-shire's gran - ite

State; Made the hills. Old New Hamp - shire, Old New

Hamp - shire, Old New Hamp - shire grand and great, We will

sing of old New Hamp - shire, Of the dear old Gran - ite ___ State.

State Song

More About New Hampshire

Books

Blohm, Craig E. *The Thirteen Colonies: New Hampshire*. San Diego, CA: Lucent Books, 2002.

Fradin, Dennis B. *The New Hampshire Colony*. Chicago: Children's Press, 1988.

Mattern, Joanne. *New Hampshire: The Granite State*. Milwaukee: World Almanac Library, 2003

Web Sites

Explore Wild New England:

http://www.wildnewengland.org

The New Hampshire Almanac:

http://www.state.nh.us/nhinfo

The Official Site of the New Hampshire Division of Travel & Tourism Development:

http://www.visitnh.gov

About the Author

Terry Allan Hicks has written books for Marshall Cavendish on subjects ranging from Ellis Island to the bald eagle. He lives with his wife, Nancy, and their sons Jamie, Jack, and Andrew in Connecticut—but he visits New Hampshire every chance he gets.

Index

Page numbers in **boldface** are illustrations.